D1703727

Selective and specific I_f inhibition in cardiovascular disease

SELECTIVE AND SPECIFIC I_f INHIBITION IN CARDIOVASCULAR DISEASE

EDITED BY
BRAMAH N. SINGH AND PAUL M. VANHOUTTE

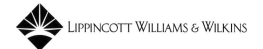

Published by Lippincott Williams & Wilkins, Third Floor, 241 Borough High Street,
London SE1 1GB, UK. Tel. +44 (0)20 7940 7500; fax. +44 (0)20 7940 7575.

Copyright © 2003 Lippincott Williams & Wilkins. All rights reserved; no part of this publication may be reproduced, stored in a retrieval system, or transmitted in any form or by any means, electronic, mechanical, photocopying, recording or otherwise without either the prior written permission of the Publisher or a licence permitting restricted copying issued in the UK by the Copyright Licensing Authority and in the USA by the Copyright Clearance Center.

Applications for permissions should be addressed to Lippincott Williams & Wilkins, 241 Borough High Street, London, SE1 1GB, UK. Fax. +44 (0)20 7940 7555.

ISBN 0-7817-4680-9

The publisher and the authors accept no responsibilities for loss incurred by any person acting or refraining from action as a result of material in or omitted from this publication.

Readers are advised that new methods and techniques described involving drug usage should be followed only in conjunction with drug manufacturers' own published literature.

Managing Editor
Isabelle Rameau
Tel: +44 (0)20 7940 7558
Editorial Project Co-ordinator
Christine Sheppard
Indexer
Merrall-Ross International Ltd

Typeset by Neil Morris, Lincolnshire, UK and printed by Jouve, France.

Customer Services can be contacted via the Lippincott Williams & Wilkins website at http://www.lww.com

This publication has been made possible through an educational grant from SERVIER

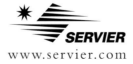

www.servier.com

CONTENTS

Contributing authors ix

INTRODUCTION
Selective and specific I_f inhibition in cardiovascular disease 1
Bramah N. Singh and Paul M. Vanhoutte

CHAPTER 1
I_f current: state of the art 3
Dario DiFrancesco

CHAPTER 2
Regulation of the cardiac pacemaker current, I_f, in normal and pathophysiological conditions 11
Jacques Lenfant and Patrick Bois

CHAPTER 3
The pacemaker current I_f in ventricular myocytes 19
Alessandro Mugelli, Laura Sartiani, Petra De Paoli, Giuseppe Lonardo, and Elisabetta Cerbai

CHAPTER 4
Molecular structure and functional expression of I_f channels from heart and central nervous system 29
Martin Biel

CHAPTER 5
Changes in heart rate and activation pathway and their role in modifying cardiac repolarization 37
Michael R. Rosen, Alexei Plotnikov, Ravil Gainullin, Parag Chandra, Bengt Herweg, and Peter Danilo Jr

CHAPTER 6
Effects of increased heart rate on coronary atherogenesis and its reversal by bradycardia induced by sinus node ablation or β-adrenergic blockade 45
Thomas B. Clarkson

CHAPTER 7
Heart rate as a risk factor in modifying the effects of myocardial ischemia: experimental and clinical correlations 53
Stephen F. Vatner

CHAPTER 8
Bradycardia and heart rate variability 61
Jean Yves Le Heuzey and Xavier Copie

CHAPTER 9
Pathophysiology of chronic and acute myocardial ischemia 69
Prediman K. Shah

CHAPTER 10
Efficacy of ivabradine in stable angina 77
Kim Fox

CHAPTER 11
Clinical interest of heart rate reduction in heart failure 85
Sergio Chierchia and Antonio Zingarelli

CHAPTER 12
Heart rate reduction and morbidity and mortality in cardiovascular disorders 95
Bramah N. Singh

References 107

Index 121

Contributing Authors

Martin Biel
Department of Pharmacy, Ludwig-Maximilians University, Munich, Germany

Patrick Bois
University of Poitiers, CNRS UMR 6558, Poitiers, France

Elisabetta Cerbai
Department of Preclinical and Clinical Pharmacology, University of Florence, Florence, Italy

Parag Chandra
Department of Pharmacology, College of Physicians and Surgeons of Columbia University, New York, NY, USA

Sergio Chierchia
Division of Cardiology, University Hospital, S. Martino, Genoa, Italy

Thomas B. Clarkson
Professor of Comparative Medicine, Comparative Medicine Clinical Research Center, Wake Forest University School of Medicine, Winston-Salem, NC, USA

Xavier Copie
Centre Cardiologique du Nord, Saint Denis, France

Peter Danilo Jr
Department of Pharmacology, College of Physicians and Surgeons of Columbia University, New York, NY, USA

Petra De Paoli
Department of Preclinical and Clinical Pharmacology, University of Florence, Florence, Italy

Dario DiFrancesco
Department of General Physiology and Biochemistry, Laboratory of Molecular Physiology and Neurobiology, University of Milan, Milan, Italy

Kim Fox
Director of Cardiology, Royal Brompton and Harefield NHS Trust, London, UK

Ravil Gainullin
Department of Pharmacology, College of Physicians and Surgeons of Columbia University, New York, NY, USA

Bengt Herweg
Department of Pharmacology, College of Physicians and Surgeons of Columbia University, New York, NY, USA

Jean Yves Le Heuzey
Department of Cardiology, Hôpital Européen Georges Pompidou, Paris, France

Jacques Lenfant
University of Poitiers, CNRS UMR 6558, Poitiers, France

Giuseppe Lonardo
Department of Preclinical and Clinical Pharmacology, University of Florence, Florence, Italy

Alessandro Mugelli
Department of Preclinical and Clinical Pharmacology, University of Florence, Florence, Italy

Alexei Plotnikov
Department of Pharmacology, College of Physicians and Surgeons of Columbia University, New York, NY, USA

Michael R. Rosen
Director, Center for Molecular Therapeutics, Departments of Pharmacology and Pediatrics, College of Physicians and Surgeons of Columbia University, New York, NY, USA

Laura Sartiani
Department of Preclinical and Clinical Pharmacology, University of Florence, Florence, Italy

Prediman K. Shah
Shapell and Webb Chair and Director, Division of Cardiology and Atherosclerosis Research Center, Cedars Sinai Medical Center, Los Angeles, CA, USA and Professor of Medicine, UCLA, Los Angeles, CA, USA

Bramah N. Singh
Professor of Medicine, Greater Los Angeles Veterans Affairs Health Care System and Department of Medicine, UCLA School of Medicine and Medical Center, Los Angeles, CA, USA

Paul M. Vanhoutte
Department of Pharmacology, Université Paris VI, Paris, France

Stephen F. Vatner
Chair, Cell Biology & Molecular Medicine, Director of Cardiovascular Research Institute, UMDNJ - New Jersey Medical School, Newark, NJ, USA

Antonio Zingarelli
Division of Cardiology, University Hospital, S. Martino, Genoa, Italy

INTRODUCTION

Selective and Specific I_f Inhibition in Cardiovascular Disease

BRAMAH N. SINGH AND PAUL M. VANHOUTTE

The data presented and discussed in this monograph support the concept of heart rate reduction as a valuable therapeutic option for reducing morbidity and mortality in a wide range of cardiovascular disease. Clinical evidence has been accumulating for many years to suggest a link between heart rate and mortality in patients with coronary artery disease (Gillum et al, 1991; Gillman et al, 1993; Habib, 1997) as well as in the general population (Habib, 2001). Epidemiologic data, particularly from the Framingham study, have also indicated a strong link between sudden cardiac death and sustained elevated heart rate, raising the issue that slow heart rate *per se* might exert an antifibrillatory action (Castelli et al, 1990; Goldberg et al, 1996). In this respect, an elevated heart rate can be considered as an independent risk factor for cardiovascular mortality. There is also evidence to suggest that a sustained elevated heart rate may play a direct role in the pathogenesis of coronary atherosclerosis (Beere et al, 1984; Perski et al, 1992). It is widely accepted that lowering heart rate can reduce the risk of cardiovascular events and increase life expectancy. The heart rate–lowering effects of β-blockers have been correlated with reduced cardiovascular and total mortality in post–myocardial infarction and heart failure patients (Kjekshus, 1986). In theory, a highly specific heart rate–lowering agent should have the same beneficial effects with respect to reduced risk and mortality and may avoid some of the drawbacks associated with β-blocker therapy.

The objectives of current therapies are to increase coronary blood flow and decrease myocardial oxygen demand. Heart rate is a critical determinant of myocardial oxygen consumption and a reduction in heart rate usually leads to a reduction in myocardial oxygen consumption. Coronary blood flow can be improved by a slower heart rate due to an increase in diastolic perfusion time during the heart cycle. The role of specific heart rate–lowering agents needs to be explored in this context. Studies so far indicate that specific heart rate–lowering agents do reduce myocardial oxygen consumption and provide significant anti-ischemic and antianginal effects with the potential for prolonging survival.

In this monograph, the epidemiology and pathophysiology of cardiovascular diseases are related to the effects of elevated heart rate and the potential benefits of heart rate reduction, with reference to the novel, specific heart rate–lowering agent ivabradine. Ivabradine (Procoralan®) selectively inhibits the hyperpolarization-activated inward I_f current in the sinoatrial node of the heart (Thollon et al, 1997), which is a major target for the physiological autonomic control of heart rate. Ivabradine induces a reduction in heart rate by decreasing the diastolic depolarization gradient and thereby reducing the spontaneous action potential firing rate of the sinoatrial node. Ivabradine is a selective and specific inhibitor of I_f with minimal effects on other cardiac currents at clinically effective doses, and the complex electrophysiology of the I_f current and its inhibition by ivabradine are discussed in detail in several chapters of this monograph. Preclinical and clinical data are also presented to enable the reader to appreciate the therapeutic potential of this promising new agent. The specific heart rate–lowering properties of ivabradine may be of value for inclusion in therapeutic regimens either in combination with or in place of currently available agents for cardiovascular diseases. Ivabradine could also be a valuable agent in exploring the benefits of selective heart rate reduction in a variety of clinical diseases with elevated heart rate.

CHAPTER 1

I_f CURRENT: STATE OF THE ART

Dario DiFrancesco

Introduction

Pacemaker activity of the heart originates in a specialized cardiac region, the sinoatrial node (SAN) in mammals or the sinus-venosus node in amphibians. Spontaneous action potentials of myocytes isolated from these natural cardiac pacemaker regions, or from other tissues able to pace, such as the atrioventricular node and from Purkinje fibers, are characterized by the presence of a particular phase of the action potential, the slow diastolic (so-called "pacemaker") depolarization (phase 4). Following an action potential, during this phase the membrane voltage slowly depolarizes, until threshold for a new action potential is reached. Thus, the slow diastolic depolarization is responsible for spontaneous activity. Early investigation aimed at describing the mechanisms responsible for pacemaker depolarization led to the proposal that a decaying K^+ current was responsible for diastolic depolarization. This idea was supported by the finding in Purkinje fibers of the so-called "pacemaker" (I_{K2}) current, which was described as a pure K^+ current activated upon depolarization in the diastolic range of voltages (Noble and Tsien, 1968). However, in the late 70s and early 80s, new evidence in Purkinje fibers and in the rabbit SAN revolutionized the K^+-decay current hypothesis. Firstly, an inward current activated on hyperpolarization ("funny" current, I_f) was discovered and shown to underlie diastolic depolarization in the rabbit SAN (Brown et al, 1979; Brown and DiFrancesco, 1980); secondly, it was demonstrated that the I_{K2} "pacemaker" current of Purkinje fibers was not a K^+ outward current activated on depolarization, but actually the opposite, that is, an inward current carried by Na^+ and K^+ and activated on hyperpolarization (DiFrancesco, 1981a,b). This demonstrated that the Purkinje fiber "pacemaker" current was the same as the SAN I_f (DiFrancesco, 1981a,b).

Starting from these early observations, investigation on the properties of the "funny" current advanced in the 1980s and 1990s to provide more detailed evidence concerning the relevance of this component to the generation of cardiac spontaneous activity and its regulation by autonomic neurotransmitters (reviewed by DiFrancesco, 1993). As well as in cardiac myocytes, hyperpolarization-activated currents (I_h currents) were described in several types of neurons, and shown to be involved in the control of cell excitability and/or spontaneous firing (see review by Pape, 1996).

More recently, various isoforms of hyperpolarization-activated, cyclic-nucleotide-gated (HCN) channels have been cloned from mammalian tissues. Heterologous expression experiments have demonstrated that HCN clones are the molecular determinants of native f/h channels (Santoro et al, 1998; Ludwig et al, 1998, 1999b; Vaccari et al, 1999; Shi et al, 1999; Ishii et al, 1999; Moroni et al, 2000).

This review briefly summarizes the present knowledge of the features of the cardiac pacemaker I_f current and its participation in the generation and modulation of pacemaker rhythm.

Basic kinetic and ionic properties of the cardiac pacemaker current

The first description of the I_f current and its relevance to pacemaker activity appeared in the late 1970s, when Brown, DiFrancesco, and Noble (1979) noticed that, in a rabbit SAN preparation, a hyperpolarization-activated current, slowly activating at voltages in the diastolic range (approximately −50 to −80 mV) could underlie the diastolic depolarization of the action potential and its acceleration by adrenaline. Following the reinterpretation of the pacemaker current in Purkinje fibers and its identification with the nodal I_f (DiFrancesco, 1981a,b), the basic ionic and kinetic properties of I_f were investigated more quantitatively in isolated SAN cells (DiFrancesco et al, 1986).

The basic properties of I_f (i.e., the activation curve, panel b, and the fully activated current-voltage (I/V) relation, panel d) for a typical rabbit SAN myocyte are shown in Figure 1.

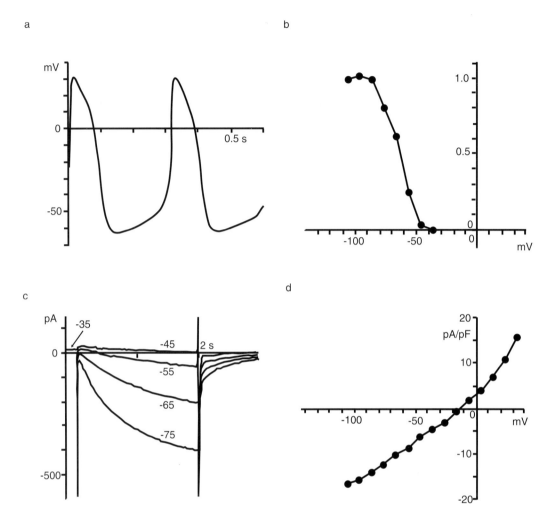

Figure 1 Properties of I_f in isolated sinoatrial node myocytes. a: spontaneous activity. b: activation curve. c: I_f records during steps to the voltages indicated. d: fully-activated I/V relation. All recordings taken at 35°C.

The range of I_f activation (Figure 1b) typically overlaps the range of diastolic depolarization of spontaneously beating pacemaker cells (compare panels a and c). Although the relevance of I_f to pacemaker depolarization has been disputed in the past based on the variability of the position of the activation curve relative to diastolic range (i.e., in some recordings I_f appears to be activated at voltages more negative than the maximum diastolic potential), evidence has accumulated showing that single-cell recordings may show a more negative I_f activation range than *in vivo* due to run-down or intracellular cyclic adenosine monophosphate (cAMP) reduction (DiFrancesco, 1991). Indeed, as is discussed below, displacement of the I_f activation curve along the voltage axis occurs naturally under the influence of internal cAMP, a mechanism representing the basis of f-channel modulation by neurotransmitters, and variability of the position of the current activation curve is expected under different experimental conditions (DiFrancesco et al, 1986; DiFrancesco and Mangoni, 1994).

Stronger arguments ruling in favor of I_f being the current mainly responsible for generation of pacemaker activity under physiological conditions rely in fact on various direct and indirect experimental observations. Among these arguments, for example, is the evidence that I_f is expressed at early but not at late stages of embryonic development in chick ventricle, and that I_f expression and spontaneous activity are correlated (Satoh and Sperelakis, 1993); f-channels are in fact also expressed in mammalian (rat) ventricle, but their voltage range of activation becomes more negative with age during neonatal development, a process that renders f-channels nonfunctional and is accompanied by a decreased membrane density and occurrence (Cerbai et al, 1999b). Further, a direct correlation between expression of pacemaker current in heart and cardiac rate has been shown using a bradycardic zebrafish mutant (Baker et al, 1997). Even more compelling evidence for a basic role of I_f in pacemaker activity comes from pharmacological evidence that reduction in I_f current due to partial block by specific blocking molecules leads to sinus node bradycardia, and that this effect can be reproduced in single cell experiments (van Bogaert and Goethals, 1987; DiFrancesco, 1994; Bois et al, 1996). Finally, the relevance of I_f-like, neuronal hyperpolarization-activated current (I_h current) to pacemaker activity has been demonstrated in several types of neurons (Pape, 1996).

The I_f activation time-constant (measured by single-exponential fitting) is about 600 ms at −70 mV (DiFrancesco and Noble, 1989), and changes steeply with voltage in the diastolic voltage range. This may represent a safety factor for limiting changes in maximum diastolic potential during activity, by allowing rapid onset of depolarization whenever the maximum diastolic potential tends to be too negative and vice versa.

As determined both in Purkinje fibers and SAN, the fully activated I/V curve of I_f is almost linear and reverses at voltages near −20 mV (in normal Tyrode solution, Figure 1d), which results from a mixed permeability of the f-channel to Na^+ and K^+ ions (DiFrancesco, 1981b; DiFrancesco et al, 1986). The mixed ionic permeability of I_f thus determines the inward ionic nature of the current in the pacemaker range of voltages, and is ultimately responsible for its depolarizing action during the diastolic phase of the action potential.

A property of I_f which is relevant to its physiological function is the increase in I_f conductance when the extracellular K^+ concentration is raised (DiFrancesco, 1981b; 1982; DiFrancesco et al, 1986). Because of the prevailing K^+ conductance during late repolarization, increasing the external K^+ concentration leads to depolarization of the maximum diastolic potential of pacing cells; since I_f activation is strongly voltage-dependent, this would tend to decrease the amount of I_f activated during diastolic depolarization, and therefore cause a substantial reduction in diastolic rate. The K^+-induced increase in I_f conductance thus compensates for the voltage-dependent decrease in current activation and reduces the bradycardic effect of hyperkalemia.

MODULATION OF CARDIAC RATE BY THE I_f CURRENT

The cardiac SAN region is the most densely innervated by the autonomic nervous system, which acts through sympathetic and parasympathetic stimuli to regulate cardiac rate. Stimulation of the sympathetic nervous system leads to β-adrenergic–mediated rate acceleration, while parasympathetic stimulation leads to muscarinic-mediated rate slowing.

Early investigation in pacemaker tissue demonstrated that rate acceleration induced by adrenaline is associated with an increase in I_f at diastolic voltages (Brown et al, 1979). Subsequent studies indicated that the adrenaline-induced I_f stimulation is due to a shift of the activation curve to more positive voltages, which increases the degree of I_f activation without altering the fully activated current, and is due to an augmented synthesis of intracellular cAMP (DiFrancesco et al, 1986). Thus, an increase in I_f due to β-adrenergic stimulation causes a faster diastolic depolarization rate and tachycardia. Low doses of β-agonists increase I_f and accelerate diastolic depolarization without changing significantly the shape and duration of the action potential (DiFrancesco, 1993), thus suggesting that the cardiac rate is controlled primarily by I_f at these low concentrations (Figure 2).

The finding that I_f mediates β-adrenergic positive chronotropism raised the obvious question as to whether I_f could also play a role in the ACh (acetylcholine)–mediated negative chronotropism. It has long been known that ACh slows cardiac rate and the spontaneous rate of isolated pacing tissue, and early studies in isolated preparations had identified an ACh-activated K^+ current ($I_{K,ACh}$) as the mechanism underlying slowing (Sakmann, Noma and Trautwein, 1983). Subsequent work indicated that ACh has an additional effect: it inhibits I_f by shifting the current activation curve to more negative voltages, a

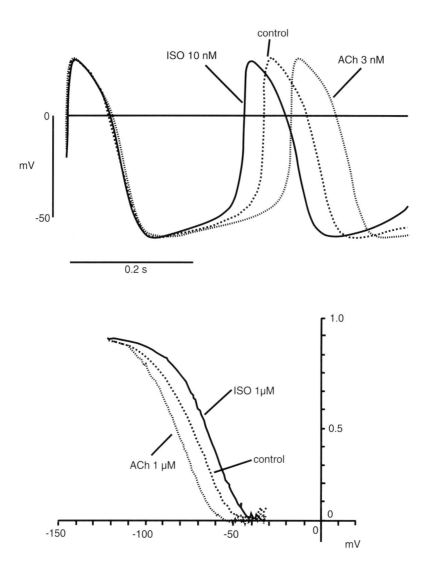

Figure 2 Top: low isoprenaline (ISO) and acetylcholine (ACh) concentrations accelerate and slow rhythm, respectively, by modifying the diastolic depolarization rate, without altering action potential shape and duration. Modified from DiFrancesco, 1993 (with permission). Bottom: actions of isoprenaline and acetylcholine on rate are mediated by I_f, whose activation curve is shifted positive (by ISO) and negative (by ACh). Modified with permission from Accili et al, 1997.

mechanism opposite to that due to catecholamines and involving G-protein–dependent inhibition of cAMP production (DiFrancesco and Tromba, 1988). Experimental evidence indeed demonstrated subsequently that the I_f reduction by ACh is a primary mechanism in the vagal-mediated chronotropic response of the heart, since the ACh concentrations inhibiting I_f and slowing spontaneous rate are some 20-fold lower than those required to activate the ACh-dependent K^+ current $I_{K,ACh}$ (DiFrancesco et al, 1989). These data are consistent with evidence that rate slowing in SAN cells due to low ACh doses occurs with a reduction in the slope of the diastolic depolarization without alteration in action potential shape and duration (Figure 2).

Thus, moderate vagal stimulation slows diastolic depolarization and heart rate by reducing intracellular cAMP and by shifting the voltage dependence of I_f activation to more negative voltages.

SINGLE f-CHANNEL RECORDING

To date, single-channel recordings of the pacemaker current have only been performed in single SAN cells (DiFrancesco, 1986; DiFrancesco and Mangoni, 1994). This limitation is possibly related to the difficulty of measuring the rather small single-channel current carried by I_f (single-channel conductance of about 1 pS). Despite the limited amount of available data, single-channel recording has allowed an understanding of the microscopic basis of I_f dual gating by negative voltage and cAMP, and of the neurotransmitter-induced I_f modulation. Thus, it has been possible to determine that the cAMP-induced current modulation is due to an increase in open channel probability which leaves unaltered the single-channel conductance (DiFrancesco, 1986); these findings are in agreement with the action of β-adrenergic stimulation in whole-cell experiments, resulting in a positive shift of the current activation curve and no modification of the fully activated I/V relation (DiFrancesco et al, 1986). Perfusion with cAMP of the intracellular side of f-channels has revealed that the action of cAMP is mediated by direct cAMP binding to the channel in the absence of protein kinase A–dependent phosphorylation, providing the first evidence that f-channels are gated by cyclic nucleotides, like cyclic nucleotide-gated (CNG) channels (DiFrancesco and Tortora, 1991), and has directly demonstrated that cAMP binding indeed results in increased single-channel open probability, with no changes in channel conductance (DiFrancesco and Mangoni, 1994).

BLOCKERS OF PACEMAKER CHANNELS

One of the properties of the pacemaker current that revealed the inward ionic nature of I_f and allowed its reinterpretation in cardiac Purkinje fibers (DiFrancesco, 1981a) is the block by cesium (Cs^+) ions (DiFrancesco, 1982). Cs^+-induced block of I_f is concentration- and voltage-dependent, with the degree of block increasing steeply at negative voltages. The voltage dependence of block can be interpreted as the result of Cs^+ ions entering the f-channel for a fraction of the electric field before binding to the blocking site. In Purkinje fibers, Cs^+ ions cross about 70% of the electric field before blocking f-channels, and the half-block concentration is 2.2 mM (DiFrancesco, 1982). In SAN cells, a similar voltage-dependent block has been reported, although the effectiveness of Cs^+ ions could be lower (DiFrancesco et al, 1986). The voltage dependence of I_f block by Cs^+ is such as to leave a substantial fraction of current available at diastolic potentials. This explains why the addition of millimolar concentrations of Cs^+ in the perfusate can slow, but cannot fully abolish, pacemaker depolarization in SAN myocytes (Denyer and Brown, 1990), and implies that Cs^+ cannot be considered as a perfect tool to dissect the contribution of I_f to diastolic depolarization.

Other substances able to act as more specific blockers of the pacemaker current have been produced more recently. These molecules are known as specific bradycardic agents (SBA) and their potential value as therapeutic agents is based on the ability to induce bradycardia without the inotropic side effects typical of other agents normally used to slow heart rate (such as calcium (Ca^{2+}) antagonists or β-blockers). It is worth noting that, because of the original misconception concerning the origin of the pacemaker depolarization and the nature of the pacemaker current (see above), SBAs were at first considered as Ca^{2+}-channel blockers (Doerr and Trautwein, 1990), and were found to be rather specific I_f blockers only later, following more careful, unbiased experimentation (van Bogaert and Goethals, 1987; DiFrancesco, 1994).

SBAs include alinidine, UL-FS49 (Figure 3), ZD-7288, and ivabradine (van Bogaert and Goethals, 1987; DiFrancesco, 1994; Gasparini and DiFrancesco, 1997; BoSmith et al, 1993; Bois et al, 1996). UL-FS49 behaves as an "open channel" blocker and inhibits f-channels in a concentration- and use-dependent way (DiFrancesco, 1994). This means that block is more efficient at more negative voltages, when more channels are open, I_f is larger, and the diastolic depolarization it generates is steeper. Thus, the bradycardic action of the drug will be more intense at greater intrinsic beating rates, that is, when it is likely to be most useful.

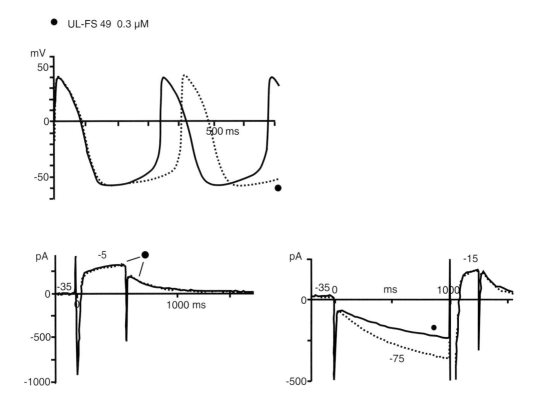

Figure 3 Action of low concentrations of a specific bradycardic agent, UL-FS 49, on ion currents in single sinoatrial node cells. Top: 0.3 µM UL-FS 49 added to normal Tyrode solution slows rate by modification of the diastolic depolarization rate only. Bottom: during steps to the voltages indicated, the same drug concentration decreases I_f (right) without modifying other time-dependent currents such as the "delayed" K+ current or the inward Ca^{2+} current (left). Temperature was 35°C.

HCN CHANNEL CLONES

Recently, molecular characterization of I_f has been possible following the cloning of a new family of cDNAs coding channels with properties similar to those of native pacemaker channels (HCNs) (Clapham, 1998; Santoro and Tibbs, 1999). The first member of this family, originally termed mBCNG1, was cloned from mouse brain (Santoro et al, 1998), and was shortly followed by cloning of other members of the family: SPIH in sea urchin (Gauss et al, 1998), mHAC1-3 (Ludwig et al, 1998), hHCN2 (Vaccari et al, 1999; Ludwig et al, 1999b), hHCN4 (Ludwig et al, 1999b), and rbHCN4 (Ishii et al, 1999) in mammals. Four different HCN isoforms (1–4) are now known (Santoro and Tibbs, 1999). As expected from the properties of native currents, HCN channels are structurally related to voltage-dependent K+ (Kv) and CNG channels: six transmembrane-domain (S1–S6), a positively charged putative voltage sensor (S4), a pore region (between S5 and S6) with a selectivity filter (GYGA) similar although not identical to that of K+ channels (GYGD), and a cyclic nucleotide binding domain at the C-terminus (Clapham, 1998). The proposed topology and functional domains of HCN channels are shown in Figure 4.

The electrophysiological properties of HCN channels expressed heterologously clearly indicate that they are the molecular determinants of native pacemaker channels in the heart and nervous system. These properties include activation on hyperpolarization, lack of deactivation, mixed permeability to Na+ and K+, voltage-dependent block by Cs+, and sensitivity to intracellular cAMP (Santoro et al, 1998; Gauss

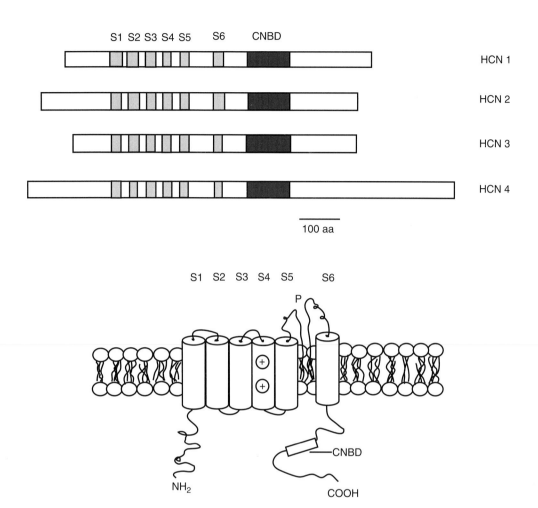

Figure 4 Top: topology of the four hyperpolarization-activated cyclic nucleotide gated (HCN) isoforms known to date. The positions of the six transmembrane and cyclic-nucleotide binding domain (CNBD) are shown. Bottom: predicted structure of HCN channels. P, pore region.

et al, 1998; Ludwig et al, 1998, 1999; Vaccari et al, 1999; Ishii et al, 1999; Moroni et al, 2000). Although qualitatively similar, kinetic and modulatory properties of different HCN isoforms differ quantitatively. Thus, for example, HCN1 has faster kinetics, and displays a reduced sensitivity to cAMP compared with HCN2 and HCN4 (Santoro and Tibbs, 1999; Ludwig et al, 1999b). Since these properties are more specifically found in neuronal than in cardiac preparations (DiFrancesco, 1993; Pape, 1996), it is interesting to verify to what extent the tissue expression of different isoforms correlates with the features of native pacemaker currents in different regions of heart and central nervous system. Indeed, a strict correlation seems to exist: thus, Northern blot analysis indicates that HCN1 is highly expressed in brain but not in whole heart, whereas HCN2 is expressed in both brain and heart (Santoro et al, 1998; Ludwig et al, 1998); also, reverse transcriptase polymerase chain reaction (RT-PCR) analysis indicates that HCN2 is expressed in atrium, ventricle, and SAN (Santoro et al, 1998). More recently, high expression of HCN4 and traces of HCN2 have been found in the rabbit SAN (Shi et al, 1999). These data suggest that HCN4 is a major determinant of the native I_f in cardiac pacemaker cells. Notably, however, HCN1 also appears to be specifically expressed in the SAN (Moroni et al, 1999).

Summary

Following its early description, the "pacemaker" I_f current, a mixed Na^+/K^+ current activated on hyperpolarization, has been extensively characterized in cardiac preparations. I_f plays a key role in the generation of diastolic depolarization and its activation is controlled, by voltage as well as by the second messenger cAMP, according to a mechanism underlying cardiac rhythm modulation by sympathetic and parasympathetic neurotransmitters. Stimulation of β-adrenergic receptors raises intracellular cAMP levels and increases I_f by a positive shift of the current activation curve, thus speeding diastolic depolarization and cardiac rate, whereas stimulation of muscarinic receptors slows rate by the opposite action.

f-channel gating by cAMP is due to direct cAMP binding to the channel protein, a property typical of CNG channels of sensory neurons. Single-channel studies have shown that f-channels have a small conductance (about 1 pS) and that cAMP increases I_f by increasing the probability of channel opening, without modifying single-channel conductance.

I_f-like currents (termed I_h) are widely expressed in several types of neurons. The properties of I_h currents are well suited to controlling neuronal excitability and the flow of information through synaptic contacts. Recently, several isoforms of HCN channels have been cloned. HCN channels belong to the superfamily of voltage-gated K^+ and CNG channels. This paves the way for novel strategies for the understanding of the molecular properties of f/h-channels.

Conclusions

In the more than 20 years since their discovery, the detailed properties of hyperpolarization-activated pacemaker channels and their functional role have been clarified for a variety of cardiac and noncardiac preparations. In heart, I_f presides over the generation and neurotransmitter-dependent modulation of the diastolic depolarization phase of the action potential of pacemaker cells. Expression of f-channels in cardiac regions other than the natural pacemaker, such as the atrioventricular node and the conduction tissue, represents a "safety" mechanism, allowing secondary pacemakers to take over and drive ventricular contraction in pathological conditions that affect normal pacemaker onset and/or propagation to the ventricles. Although expression of f-channels in ventricular muscle is nonfunctional in the adult, it may have an important functional role at early stages during development. It will be interesting to understand what the role of increased I_f expression in hypertrophic ventricle actually is.

f-like hyperpolarization-activated pacemaker channels (h-channels) are also expressed in a large variety of neuronal types. In general, their role is to control neuronal excitability or, in neurons where spontaneous firing occurs, to modulate firing rate, but new evidence is being gathered which indicates that h-channels may have a previously unsuspected function in controlling synaptic efficiency.

The molecular characterization of pacemaker channels has received a strong impulse with the cloning of HCN channels. This allows the structural basis of ionic, kinetic, and modulatory properties of native f/h channels to be investigated by the use of site-directed mutagenesis and patch-clamp analysis. A molecular-biological approach can also be used to gain information about possible correlations between naturally occurring mutations in the primary sequence of HCN channels and pathological alterations of pacemaker and excitability properties in the heart. Finally, knowledge of the structure–function relationship of HCN channel clones will allow new drugs to be developed, which will have specific binding sites on the channels as their target, and which will also therefore be able to modify channel function more specifically, a possibility that may have significant clinical implications in the treatment of cardiovascular disorders.

Acknowledgments

Part of the most recent work reviewed here was supported by Telethon (grant 971) and MURST (Cofin 1999).

CHAPTER 2

REGULATION OF THE CARDIAC PACEMAKER CURRENT, I_f, IN NORMAL AND PATHOPHYSIOLOGICAL CONDITIONS

JACQUES LENFANT AND PATRICK BOIS

INTRODUCTION

Cardiac pacemaker activity originates in specialized sinoatrial (SA) node myocytes that are characterized by the ability to beat spontaneously. The rhythmic activity of the SA node cells results from a typical phase of the action potential, slow diastolic depolarization. During this phase, corresponding to diastole of the cardiac contraction cycle, the membrane slowly depolarizes following termination of an action potential until the threshold for a new action potential is reached. Among the ionic mechanisms involved in the diastolic depolarization, the pacemaker current, I_f, is the major component contributing to the initiation of this phase and to the modulation of its slope in response to the autonomic neurotransmitters controlling cardiac rate (DiFrancesco, 1993).

The aim of this chapter is to critically discuss the involvement of the pacemaker current in the modulation of cardiac rhythm by different signaling mechanisms in normal and pathophysiological situations.

REGULATION OF THE PACEMAKER CURRENT BY THE AUTONOMIC NERVOUS SYSTEM

Neurotransmitters

Besides generating the spontaneous activity of SA node cells, diastolic depolarization is involved in the control of cardiac rate by autonomic neurotransmitters. Under normal conditions, low doses of neurotransmitters modify the rhythmic activity of SA node cells by changing the steepness of the slow depolarization phase. In this case, changes in frequency occur with little modification of the shape and duration of the action potential and I_f is considered to be the main target of neurotransmitters, since the background current and $I_{Ca,T}$, the other ionic mechanisms involved in the diastolic depolarization, are insensitive to β-adrenergic and muscarinic stimulation (DiFrancesco, 1993). Furthermore, larger rhythm modifications imply the modulation of other ionic mechanisms, such as $I_{Ca,L}$ and I_K and consequent changes in the shape of the action potential.

The participation of I_f in the autonomic control of cardiac rate can be described as follows: catecholamines increase I_f by stimulating adenylyl cyclase activity and cyclic adenosine monophosphate (cAMP) production, via β-adrenoceptors coupled with guanine nucleotide-binding (G_s) proteins. Direct action of cAMP on f-channels results in a positive shift of the f-current activation curve, thus more current is available to drive the process of diastolic depolarization which accelerates this phase and, hence, spontaneous activity. Acetylcholine decreases I_f and consequently the cardiac rate, by reducing adenylyl cyclase activity and cAMP production via the stimulation of muscarinic receptors coupled with G_i proteins, leading to a negative shift of the I_f activation curve (DiFrancesco, 1993).

In addition to the direct effect of cAMP, f-channels are directly controlled by G proteins, which may account for the ability of the autonomic nervous system to produce a rapid effect within a single heart beat (Yatani et al, 1990). Although controls of f-current by cAMP and G proteins are not mutually incompatible, several observations are in favor of a direct modulation of I_f mainly by cAMP. In SA node cells isolated from rabbit heart, the effect of acetylcholine has been compared, in different configurations of a patch-clamp, on I_f and on an acetylcholine-activated potassium current, $I_{K(ACh)}$, known to be specifically activated via a direct G protein mechanism. In whole cell configuration, I_f responded to acetylcholine more slowly than $I_{K(ACh)}$, consistent with a cAMP-dependent cytoplasmic pathway (Accili et al, 1998). In cell-attached conditions where cytoplasmic substrates were present, acetylcholine added to the external solution depressed I_f but never induced change in $I_{K(ACh)}$, recorded in the membrane delimited mode. In the outside-out configuration, where cytoplasmic substrates were completely dialyzed, acetylcholine activated $I_{K(ACh)}$ but had no effect on I_f (Renaudon et al, 1997). From these results, it can be concluded that the regulation of I_f by muscarinic receptors does not involve a direct G protein pathway.

While there is general agreement that the modulation of f-current by neurotransmitters is mediated by adenylyl cyclase activity, it is still a matter of debate whether direct cAMP binding or phosphorylation by cAMP-dependent protein kinase A (PKA) is the main mechanism involved. While a direct action of cAMP on f-channels has been demonstrated in SA node cells (DiFrancesco and Tortora, 1991), phosphorylation of f-channels via PKA has been reported in Purkinje cells (Chang et al, 1991). In murine embryonic stem cell-derived cardiomyocytes, known to recapitulate cardiomyogenesis *in vitro*, I_f is functionally expressed during early stages of development and displays similar biophysical characteristics to those reported for terminally differentiated cardiomyocytes. At these early stages, the activation of f-channels appears to be mediated by phosphorylation via PKA rather than by direct cAMP binding. It remains to be examined whether, during postnatal development, the switch towards a specifically direct cAMP-mediated stimulation of I_f occurs and whether this is related to different types of f-channels (Abi-Gerges et al, 2000).

Endogenous peptides

In addition to the classic neurotransmitters, small active peptides also exist in the autonomic nervous system. Two peptides, vasoactive intestinal peptide (VIP) and neuropeptide Y (NPY), are colocalized with neurotransmitters in the nerve endings of cardiac tissue (Lundberg and Hökfelt, 1986). The effects of VIP and NPY have been investigated on the pacemaker current in Purkinje fibers, by means of a two-microelectrode voltage-clamp technique. VIP reversibly increases and NPY decreases I_f elicited by a hyperpolarizing pulse. Peptides act on the f-current by shifting its activation curve on the voltage axis in a positive or negative direction, without modifying maximal conductance of f-channels. The response of I_f to VIP or NPY is mediated through the positive or negative alteration of adenylyl cyclase activity and consequently through changes in cAMP levels (Chang et al, 1994). A similar mode of action of VIP has been reported in SA node cells, by using a patch-clamp method. As shown in Figure 1, the peptide reversibly increases I_f. It accelerates the spontaneous activity of the cell by increasing the slope of the diastolic depolarization phase, in agreement with a rise in I_f (Accili et al, 1996). In the cardiac nervous system, VIP coexists with acetylcholine in parasympathetic endings whereas NPY is costored with catecholamines in sympathetic nerve terminals. Two types of subcellular storage sites are present in nerve endings: small clear sites contain classic transmitters and larger dense-core vesicles contain peptides and classic transmitters. The release of the two types of vesicles is differentially regulated by the frequency of nervous stimulation. In response to low or normal firing rates, there are only small amounts of classic neurotransmitters released from clear vesicles. In higher or longer-lasting nervous stimulation, the two types of storage sites release peptides and transmitters (Lundberg and Hökfelt, 1986). As peptides and neurotransmitters colocalized in the same nerve endings have opposite actions on I_f, the role of peptides could be to reduce the excessive effects of transmitters on the heart rate (Chang et al, 1994).

Other peptides seem to be localized in the autonomic nervous system (e.g., atrial natriuretic peptide, C-type natriuretic peptide). It is clear that the nervous system is not simply restricted to adrenergic or cholinergic transmission. It is capable of a fine tuning in the control of heart rate, partly via the modulation of the pacemaker current. Further investigations are needed to detail the functional significance of these various peptide effects.

REGULATION OF THE PACEMAKER CURRENT THROUGH OTHER SIGNALING PATHWAYS

Adenosine

Among local modulating factors controlling cardiac function, the nucleoside adenosine has a central role. It is released from heart cells and can rise greatly under the action of β-agonists during increases in heart work as well as during cardiac ischemia. Adenosine is known to stabilize excessive positive chronotropic effects induced by adrenergic stimulation, but it can reduce automaticity in SA node cells under basal conditions,

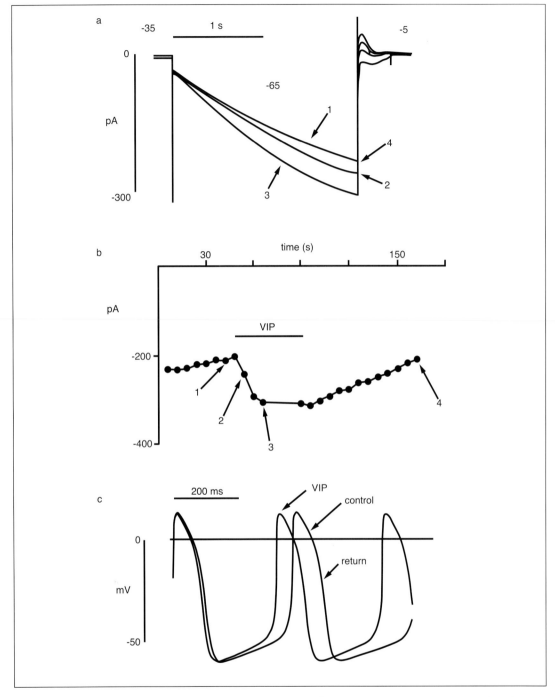

Figure 1 Effect of vasoactive intestinal peptide (VIP) on I_f and on spontaneous rate in sinoatrial node cells. a: In whole-cell configuration, hyperpolarizing steps to –65 mV, from a holding potential of –35 mV, were applied every 6 s to elicit I_f before (1), during (2–3), and after (4) perfusion with VIP. In this cell, I_f increased during exposure to VIP and returned toward control levels after VIP removal. b: Time course of I_f amplitude at –65 mV for the same cell. c: Spontaneous activity recorded in an unclamped cell. During the perfusion with VIP, the frequency is increased by 14%. Reproduced with permission from Accili et al, 1996 © 1996 Springer-Verlag.

by activating specific potassium channels (Belardinelli et al, 1988). In these cells, adenosine also reduces basal I_f by shifting its activation curve towards more negative potential values. Adenosine exerts local modulation of sinus rate through signaling pathways similar to those used by acetylcholine (Zaza et al, 1996).

A current with the characteristics of I_f is present in human isolated atrial myocytes. The voltage range of its activation does not support a functional role under physiological conditions but its properties can be modulated by disease in such a way that it may be implicated in initiating atrial arrhythmias. The stimulation of A_1-adenosine receptors by a selective agonist (cyclopentyladenosine) in human atrial cells reduces basal I_f in the same way as in SA node myocytes (Porciatti et al, 1997). The contribution of negative chronotropic effects of adenosine on human atrial activity in pathological conditions remains to be explored.

Nitric oxide

Nitric oxide (NO) is an important second messenger implicated in mediating the action of various neurotransmitters in many tissues including the cardiovascular system. The systemic administration of NO donors (such as sodium nitroprusside) is associated with an increase in heart rate, due to a neurally mediated reflex response to the fall in arterial blood pressure (Chen et al, 1982). However, NO donors can stimulate SA node activity independent of the arterial baroreflex. In spontaneously beating SA node/atrial preparations isolated from guinea pig heart, NO donors modulate rhythmic activity in a concentration-dependent biphasic fashion, with a gradual increase in beating rate at low concentrations and a reduction at high concentrations (Musialek et al, 1997). Direct recordings in rabbit SA node cells show that I_f in the basal state increases when NO donors are applied (Musialek et al, 1997; Yoo et al, 1998) but decreases when it is first stimulated by isoproterenol, a β-adrenoceptor agonist (Yoo et al, 1998). Both effects are abolished by a guanylyl cyclase inhibitor suggesting that the action of NO is mediated by cyclic guanosine monophosphate (cGMP). The dual effect of NO on I_f can be explained as follows (Yoo et al, 1998): the inhibitory effect is mediated by the breakdown of cAMP via the activation of cGMP-stimulated phosphodiesterase; the stimulatory effect can be attributable to direct binding of cGMP to f-channels since this nucleotide can increase I_f in the same way as cAMP but with a lower potency (DiFrancesco and Tortora, 1991).

Thyroid hormones

The cardiovascular system is a major target for thyroid hormone action. In hyperthyroidism, the main cardiac manifestation is an increase in resting heart rate with a high marked degree of sinus tachycardia, resulting in a rise in cardiac output and contractility (Klein and Ojamaa, 1998). Two concepts have been put forward to explain how thyroid hormones exert their cardiac effects. First, they interact with the sympathetic nervous system by enhancing responsiveness to sympathetic stimulation by modulating adrenergic receptor function or density (Bahouth et al, 1997). Second, thyroid hormones have direct effects on cardiac myocytes by the stimulation of specific nuclear receptors influencing mRNA expression of ionic channel genes, such as those of voltage-gated potassium channels (Sun et al, 2000). Thyroid hormones can also modulate the pacemaker current by an intracellular mechanism independent of sympathetic stimulation. In SA node cells from the rabbit heart, the effect of triiodothyronine (T_3) has been investigated on I_f, using the patch-clamp technique in whole cell configuration. In cells incubated for several hours (5–7 h) in a medium containing T_3, the hormone significantly increases I_f whereas reverse T_3, the inactive form of T_3, used in the same conditions, has no effect on the pacemaker current (Figure 2). The hormone increases I_f by raising the maximal conductance without inducing a shift of the activation curve. Intracellular levels of cAMP are not modified by the hormone, since isoprenaline, a β-adrenergic agonist, is still able to increase I_f by a positive shift of the activation curve in T_3-treated cells (Renaudon et al, 2000).

Four isoforms of the f-channel have been cloned, HCN1-4 (Hyperpolarization-activated Cyclic Nucleotide-gated channels) and their functional properties have been characterized (Ludwig et al, 1998; Santoro et al, 1998). In rat myocardium in different thyroidal states, the analysis of HCN2 mRNA by Northern blotting shows a significant positive effect of thyroid hormone on HCN2 expression (Pachucki et al, 1999). In mice with complete elimination of receptor genes for T_3, bradycardia occurs linked to decreased levels of HCN2 and HCN4 gene expression (Gloss et al, 2001). These results suggest that the acceleration of heart rate with hyperthyroidism is the consequence of a stimulation of f-channel

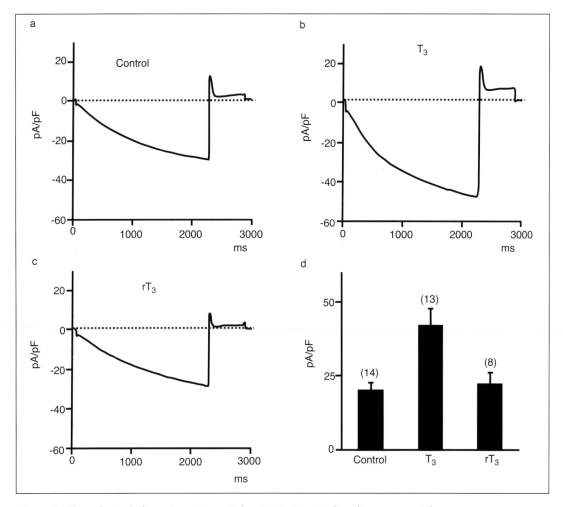

Figure 2 Effect of triiodothyronine (T_3) on I_f density in sinoatrial node myocytes. The current was recorded during a 2.2 s hyperpolarizing step of −90 mV induced from a holding potential of −35 mV followed by a step to +20 mV. a–c: examples of current traces recorded from untreated cell (a), T_3-treated cell (b) and reverse T_3-treated cell (c). d: Bar graphs representing the average of I_f density values in untreated cells, in T_3- and reverse (r)T_3-treated cells. In each condition, cells were incubated for 5–7 h before measurement of f-current. Number of cells is given in parentheses. In cells incubated with T_3, the mean values of I_f density are increased by about 110%. Reproduced with permission from Renaudon et al, 2000 © 2000 Overseas Publishers Association.

transcription, leading to an increase in I_f. It should be of interest to analyze the consequence of hyperthyroidism on the expression of HCN1 and HCN4 that are the dominant HCN transcripts in SA node myocytes (Shi et al, 1999). Overexpression of these genes may be involved in the sinus tachycardia observed in hyperthyroidism. In addition, the pacemaker current can be enhanced through the T_3-induced upregulation of β-adrenergic receptors.

THE PACEMAKER CURRENT, A TARGET FOR SPECIFIC HEART RATE–LOWERING AGENTS

In the presence of a restricted coronary blood supply to the heart, an increase in beating rate is an important factor contributing to myocardial ischemia. For this reason, pharmacological tools such as

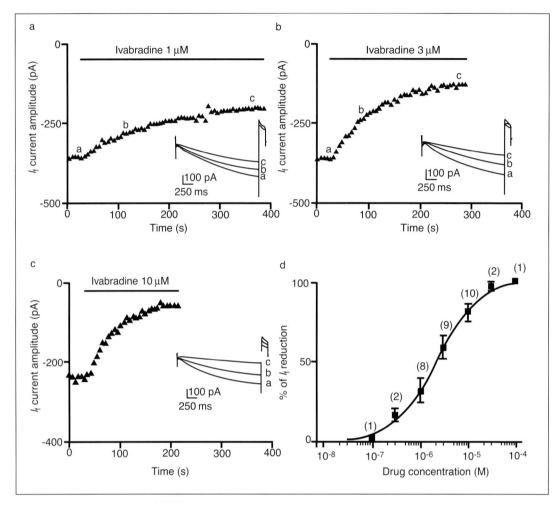

Figure 3 Use-dependent block of I_f by ivabradine at 1 µM (a), 3 µM (b), and 10 µM (c), in SA node cells. In whole-cell configuration, the current was elicited by hyperpolarizing steps to –100 mV from a holding potential of –30 mV. The graphs plot the amplitude of the current which was taken as the difference between final and initial current, before and during cell perfusion with ivabradine. The inset figures show a set of three I_f traces recorded in sequence before (a) and during cell perfusion with ivabradine (b–c). d: Graph showing a concentration-response curve for use-dependent block of I_f by ivabradine. The estimated value of IC_{50} is 2.18 µM. Number of cells is indicated above each point of the curve. Modified with permission from Bois et al, 1996.

β-blockers or some calcium channel blockers (such as diltiazem and verapamil) able to reduce heart rate are used for the treatment of ischemia. However, these agents may exert concomitant negative inotropic and hypotensive effects, which are potentially deleterious during ischemia. A novel class of pharmacological substances is reputed to induce sinus bradycardia without additional hemodynamic effects (Kobinger and Lillie, 1987). Ivabradine and zatebradine are the most potent heart rate–lowering agents of this class. They slow the rhythmic activity of pacemaker cells via an inhibition of I_f. In SA node cells from rabbit heart, ivabradine induces a marked exponential use-dependent blockade of f-current without shift of the voltage range of its activation curve. The rate of blockade increases with the drug concentration (Figure 3). The presence of a use-dependent effect of ivabradine on I_f indicates that the agent has an affinity for the open state of f-channels (Bois et al, 1996). Similar effects of zatebradine on the pacemaker current are observed in the same preparation (Goethals et al, 1993). However, a comparative study of the

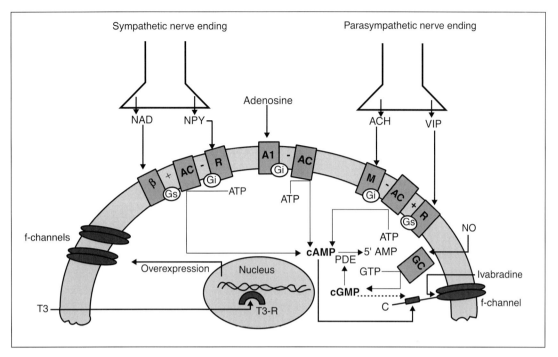

Figure 4 Schematic representation of the main signaling pathways involved in the regulation of I_f in a sinoatrial node cell. β, adrenergic receptor; A1, adenosine receptor; AC, adenylyl cyclase; ACH, acetylcholine; AMP, adenosine monophosphate; ATP, adenosine triphosphate; cAMP, cyclic adenosine monophosphate; cGMP, cyclic guanosine monophosphate; GC, guanylyl cyclase; GTP, guanosine triphosphate; M, muscarinic receptor; NAD, nicotinamide adenine dinucleotide; NO, nitric oxide; NPY, neuropeptide Y; PDE, phosphodiesterase; R, NPY or VIP receptor; T3, triiodothyronine; T3-R, triiodothyronine receptor; VIP, vasoactive intestinal peptide.

selective effect of the two agents on I_f shows that zatebradine can also reduce the delayed outward potassium current at concentrations where ivabradine has no effect on this current (Bois et al, 1996). A reduction in the delayed outward current prolongs the action potential duration which, associated with a slowing of the heart rate, can induce early after-depolarizations known to be a cause of polymorphic ventricular tachyarrhythmias (Thollon et al, 1994).

Conclusion

Figure 4 gives a schematic view of the main signaling pathways involved in the regulation of the pacemaker current in myocytes of the SA node. Under physiological conditions, low doses of the neurotransmitters acetylcholine and noradrenaline control heart rate by mainly modulating the pacemaker current of SA node cells, through changes in cAMP that interacts with its cytoplasmic binding site localized in the carboxy-terminus of the f-channel protein. With higher doses of neurotransmitters, $I_{Ca,L}$ and I_K are also affected by changes in the phosphorylation of their channels through kinase A activity (not shown in Figure 4). In this case, coreleased peptides VIP and NPY can reduce an excessive effect of neurotransmitters on the three ionic mechanisms. Adenosine reduces I_f via the stimulation of its A_1-receptors, with effects comparable to those of acetylcholine. The local action of adenosine in SA node cells may lead to a negative feedback control of sinus rate during physiological metabolic stress (Zaza et al, 1996). NO stimulates cGMP-dependent pathways by binding to the cytosolic form of guanylyl cyclase. Its positive chronotropic effect through a direct binding of cGMP on f-channels has to be related to low basal levels of cAMP, since cGMP is less potent than cAMP in activating I_f (DiFrancesco and Tortora, 1991). The stimulation of the pacemaker current by endogenous NO may be implicated in the sinus tachycardia that accompanies pathological conditions associated with myocardial production of NO.

Although f-current is the main ionic mechanism involved in the genesis and regulation of the spontaneous activity of SA node cells in physiological conditions, overexpression of f-channels can be observed in pathological situations such as thyrotoxicosis leading to sinus tachycardia. The involvement of the f-current can be reduced by using specific heart rate–lowering agents such as ivabradine. After having passed the cell membrane, the molecule seems to reach a binding site located inside the pore of the f-channel, which remains to be characterized. Overexpression of f-channels is also observed in ventricular cells from hypertrophied mammalian heart (Cerbai et al, 1994b; Farès et al, 1998) and from human failing heart (Cerbai et al, 1997). Under these pathological conditions, I_f could interact with other mechanisms and thus contribute to the appearance of ventricular arrhythmias. As the presence of cloned HCN channels in different types of heart myocytes is compatible with the characteristics of I_f observed in these cells (Ludwig et al, 1999a), the differential expression of the genes offers the possibility of developing other therapeutic agents that would target regionally specific f-channels for the prevention and treatment of cardiac arrhythmias.

Finally, the regulation of the f-channel function by neurotransmitters and other signaling mechanisms is the key process in controlling heart rate under normal conditions, and I_f is a promising target for a direct pharmacological control of cardiac frequency in the treatment of heart diseases.

CHAPTER 3

THE PACEMAKER CURRENT I_f IN VENTRICULAR MYOCYTES

ALESSANDRO MUGELLI, LAURA SARTIANI, PETRA DE PAOLI,
GIUSEPPE LONARDO, AND ELISABETTA CERBAI

INTRODUCTION

During hypertrophy and failure, cardiac myocytes change their phenotype with marked enlargement in their size (Gerdes et al, 1996). This is associated with deterioration in contractile function (affecting both contraction and relaxation phases and responses to catecholamines) (Davies et al, 1995), and induction of a specific gene program involving several groups of genes (Swynghedauw, 1999; Chien, 1999). These include genes encoding sarcomeric and cytoskeletal proteins, calcium handling proteins, ion channels, metabolic enzymes, secreted cytokines and growth factors, and enzymes involved in the apoptotic pathway. One of the major consequences is the modification in the electrophysiological properties of cardiomyocytes (Tomaselli and Marban, 1999). The functional changes in the activity of different ion channels, transporters, and receptors are likely to predispose to cardiac arrhythmias, which remain an important cause of death in patients with myocardial failure. In fact, despite optimal medical treatment, the prognosis of heart failure remains poor with over 15% of patients dying within one year after diagnosis and with a mortality greater than 80% after six years (Konstam and Remme, 1998). Up to 50% of the deaths are sudden and unexpected (Konstam and Remme, 1998).

Prolongation of action potential duration (see Tomaselli and Marban, 1999 for a review) has been found both in tissues and cells isolated from the ventricles of animals with hypertrophy and heart failure as well as in ventricular tissues and cells from failing human hearts. Prolongation of the repolarization phase has been generally considered as the main arrhythmogenic alteration in heart failure (Tomaselli et al, 1994). This phenomenon appears to be due to a selective reduction in the transient outward current I_{to}, and has been clearly documented both in myocytes isolated from old spontaneous hypertensive rats (SHR) (Cerbai et al, 1994a) and in myocytes isolated from the failing human heart (Beuckelmann et al, 1993; Nabauer et al, 1993; Tomaselli et al, 1994).

A current having the characteristics of the pacemaker current I_f, which underlies diastolic depolarization in pacemaker cells (DiFrancesco, 1993), is present in hypertrophied or failing ventricular myocytes. In this chapter, the properties of the pacemaker current expressed in ventricular myocytes isolated from animal models of hypertrophy and failure and from human failing hearts will be reviewed and its significance in arrhythmogenesis will be discussed.

THE PACEMAKER CURRENT I_f IN HYPERTROPHIED RAT VENTRICULAR MYOCYTES

The development of myocardial hypertrophy in response to chronic pressure overload is a complex adaptive phenomenon and a predictor of the progression to cardiac failure (Levy et al, 1996). SHR are a suitable animal model, which is predictive of the alterations occurring in human cardiac hypertrophy and failure and widely used for studying the progression from compensated hypertrophy to overt failure (Bing et al, 1995). SHR develop left ventricular hypertrophy in response to pressure overload through a process that evolves continuously during life. At 18 months of age, SHR show severe compensated left ventricular hypertrophy and, between the ages of 18 and 24 months, 57% of male SHR have evidence of cardiac failure. In old (18-month-old) SHR, the action potential duration is prolonged (Figure 1 a, b) due to a decrease in the repolarizing transient outward current density (Cerbai et al, 1994a); a similar alteration has been observed in failing human myocytes (Beuckelmann et al, 1993; Tomaselli et al, 1994). Moreover,

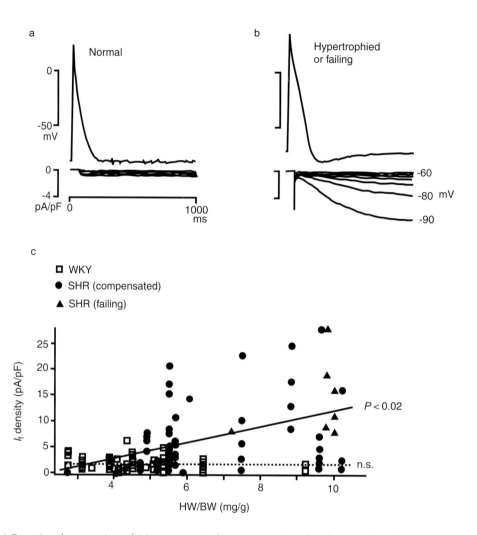

Figure 1 Functional expression of I_f in rat ventricular myocytes is related to cardiac disease. Recordings from patch-clamp experiments in the whole-cell configuration, performed in single cells enzymatically isolated from the left ventricle of control (a) and hypertrophied or failing rat hearts (b). Upper traces of panel a and b show typical action potentials recorded in current-clamp mode, in cells superfused with control Tyrode's solution. Note the diastolic depolarization phase in the hypertrophied myocyte. Bottom traces are recorded in voltage-clamp mode during increasingly negative steps, in cells superfused with a modified Tyrode's solution (containing $BaCl_2$, $MnCl_2$, and 4-aminopyridine in order to block overlapping currents and high KCl concentration to amplify the current). While current traces are completely flat in normal cells, a time-dependent exponentially activating current, whose properties resemble those of I_f, is present in more than 90% of the hypertrophied myocytes (panel b). Current amplitude measured at –120 mV was normalized to cell size (membrane capacitance), expressed in picoAmpere/picoFarad and plotted as a function of the degree of myocardial hypertrophy (HW/BW). Panel c shows the results of such an analysis: in hypertensive rats (SHR), the progression from moderate to severe compensated hypertrophy (SHR compensated, closed circles) and finally to decompensated hypertrophy (SHR failing, closed triangles) is accompanied by a parallel increase in current density, which is therefore significantly related to the heart weight to body weight ratio (HW/BW). A similar relation is not present in control nonhypertensive animals (Wistar-Kyoto [WKY]) during aging (dotted line, not significant).

left ventricular myocytes from old SHR with severe myocardial hypertrophy and/or failure show a marked diastolic depolarization phase due to overexpression of the pacemaker channel I_f (Cerbai et al,

1994b; Cerbai et al, 1995; Cerbai et al, 1996). I_f was present in the majority of myocytes isolated from old SHR, while in the majority of normal ventricular myocytes no time-dependent current was recorded upon hyperpolarization (Figure 1 a, b). When present, the current activated at about −70 mV and the voltage of half-maximal activation was −85 mV.

The presence of I_f was associated with the presence of a diastolic depolarization phase. I_f expression did not depend on cell size, as suggested by the lack of correlation between I_f amplitude and cell capacitance (an index of cell dimension). However, its density (amplitude normalized to cell size) was linearly related to the severity of hypertrophy (expressed by the ratio HW/BW) in SHR; I_f density was even greater in myocytes isolated from the heart of rats having signs of heart failure (Figure 1c). Such a relationship was not present in normotensive rats (Wistar Kyoto [WKY]), suggesting that the disease is important in the development of the phenomenon.

HYPERTROPHY INDUCES RE-EXPRESSION OF I_f

As previously stated, hypertrophy induces re-expression of genes encoding fetal proteins. Thus, the possibility exists that hypertrophy may induce the re-expression of a current, which, like I_f, is already present during fetal life. In fact, an I_f-like current has been recorded in spontaneously beating embryonic or neonatal ventricular myocytes (Brochu et al, 1992; Robinson et al, 1997; Yasui et al, 2001). Developmental changes in neonatal rat ventricular cells are characterized by a significant increase in the density of the transient outward current I_{to} and by the hypertrophy of myocytes (Kilborn and Fedida, 1990).

A better understanding of the changes in the electrophysiological properties of I_f throughout postnatal development of ventricular myocytes which, in the adult stage, are physiologically quiescent and do not express I_f (Cerbai et al, 1996), is important for an in-depth comprehension of the mechanisms and factors leading to and controlling its reappearance during disease (ie, hypertrophy and failure). I_f is expressed in ventricular myocytes isolated from newborn rats: the current occurred in all myocytes and its density was maximal at one to two days after birth, progressively decreasing during development (Figure 2).

Two weeks after birth, fewer than half of the myocytes expressed I_f, which when present was of small amplitude. Only one third of myocytes isolated from the hearts of rats at four weeks of age expressed I_f, which was of very small amplitude. During the same period of time, action potential duration progressively shortened, assuming the typical profile of the adult type. Thus, I_f is expressed in rat ventricular myocytes immediately after birth (Brochu et al, 1992; Cerbai et al, 1999b; Robinson et al, 1997) and likely during fetal life (Yasui et al, 2001); it almost disappears with development, and is re-expressed during severe hypertrophy (Cerbai et al, 1996) and failure (Cerbai et al, 1995; Cerbai et al, 1997). In other words, the behavior of I_f during natural cell growth is opposite to that during pathological hypertrophy. Disappearance of I_f in ventricular myocytes during early development occurs while the cell size increases as postnatal cellular growth develops. During pathological hypertrophy, both cell size and I_f density increase. Changes in I_f density during postnatal development, and in normal or diseased aging are shown in Figure 3a.

Thus, it appears that it is not the cellular growth per se which triggers the phenomenon, but other factors must be involved. This is not surprising, since the modification of the electrophysiological properties (i.e., changes in I_{to}) may be different during the hypertrophic process. During cell growth in neonatal cells, I_{to} increases (Guo et al, 1996; Kilborn and Fedida, 1990), while during hypertrophy due to pressure overload (Cerbai et al, 1994a) or following myocardial infarction (Aimond et al, 1999) I_{to} decreases. Changes in I_{to} density during postnatal development, and normal or diseased aging are shown in Figure 3b. Furthermore, cell growth and expression of I_{to} are independently regulated by serum factors and thyroid hormone (Guo et al, 1996; Guo et al, 1998; Shimoni et al, 1997). In neonatal ventricular myocytes cultured in serum-free conditions, basic fibroblast growth factor promotes I_{to} expression without a concomitant increase in cell size (Guo et al, 1996). In the same cells, well-known hypertrophic agents such as phenylephrine and endothelin-1 suppress the expression of the Kv 4.2 α-subunit (one of

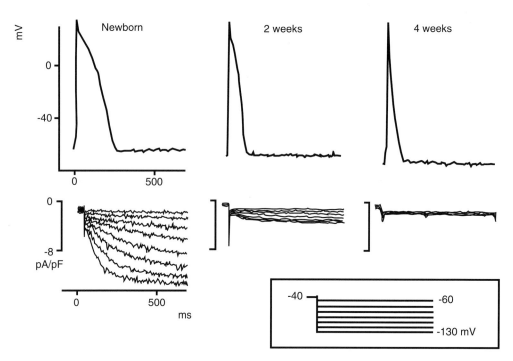

Figure 2 Postnatal electrophysiological changes in rat ventricular myocytes. Action potentials and I_f were recorded in ventricular myocytes enzymatically isolated from the heart of newborn rats, and of 2 and 4 weeks of age, using an experimental approach similar to that described in Figure 1 for adult myocytes. The duration of the action potential progressively shortens during maturation as a result of increasing potassium outward currents. Also, the diastolic depolarization, which is present in newborn rat cells, disappeared thereafter: this phenomenon is accompanied by a clear-cut decrease in the density of the pacemaker current I_f, as demonstrated by the recordings shown in bottom panels. Each of these panels shows currents activated upon hyperpolarization (see the voltage protocol in the inset): an increasing inward current is evident in newborn cells, it is still discernible at two weeks even though it has a smaller density, but current traces are flat at four weeks, an age at which the electrophysiological maturation of the heart is complete.

the isoforms whose proteins largely accounts for I_{to} in the "mature" ventricular rat cell and is upregulated during postnatal development), while producing a clear-cut increase in cell size (Guo et al, 1998). On the whole, a variety of stimuli may specifically promote or inhibit the expression of genes encoding channel proteins, this action being concomitant with or independent from the activation of cell growth. In line with this is the observation (Cerbai et al, 2000) that angiotensin II plays a major role in controlling the expression of both I_{to} and I_f. Chronic AT_1 receptor blockade with losartan in old SHR prevents in fact not only the development of myocyte hypertrophy, but also the associated electrophysiological alterations, that is, the decrease in I_{to} and the increase in I_f.

MODULATION BY β-ADRENOCEPTOR STIMULATION

A diminished response to β-adrenergic stimulation has been consistently found in the human failing heart (for a review, see Post et al, 1999). Similar modifications have been observed in hypertrophied ventricular myocytes from hypertensive (Scamps et al, 1990) and infarcted rat hearts (Aimond et al, 1999). This phenomenon has been attributed to the development of several signal transduction defects in the β-adrenoceptor (AR) pathway, such as the downregulation of β-adrenoceptor and the upregulation of

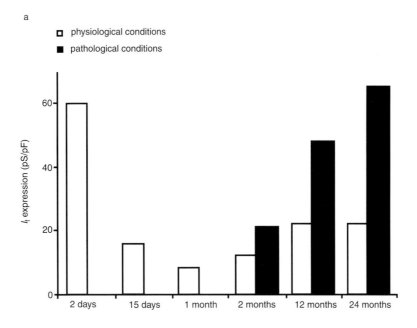

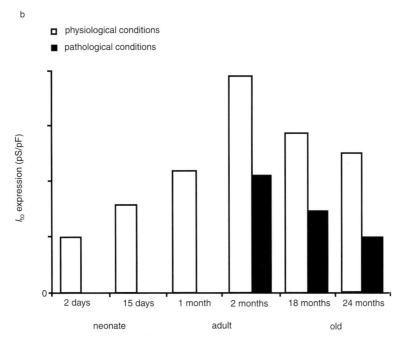

Figure 3 Age-dependent expression of cardiac channels in physiological and pathological conditions. Expression of I_f (a) and I_{to} (b) undergoes opposite changes during postnatal development and aging: in rat ventricular myocytes, during the first month of life, I_f density decreases and I_{to} density increases (Cerbai et al, 1999b; Guo et al, 1996). Physiological aging is associated with little changes (I_f) or a small reduction (I_{to}) in current density (white columns). However, in cardiac disease such as hypertrophy and failure (black columns), cellular electrophysiological properties reverse toward a neonatal phenotype, distinguished by marked over-expression of I_f (a) and downregulation of I_{to} (b) (Cerbai et al, 1994a; Cerbai et al, 1995; Cerbai et al, 1996; Aimond et al, 1999).

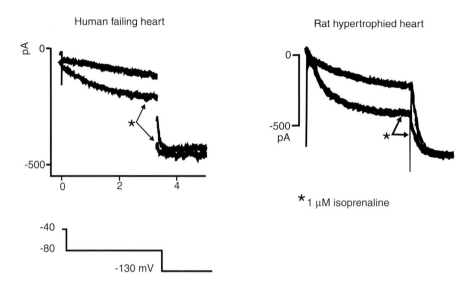

Figure 4 β-Adrenoceptor modulation of ventricular f channels. The effect of β-adrenoceptor stimulation has been tested in both human and rat ventricular myocytes expressing I_f. Human myocytes were isolated from explanted failing hearts by perfusing with the enzymatic solution a small portion of the left ventricle through a branch of a visible coronary artery. The f-current was recorded by using extracellular solutions similar to those already described for hypertrophied rat myocytes. Each panel shows superimposed current traces recorded using the two-step protocol shown in the bottom, before and after superfusion with 1 µM isoprenaline (arrows). β-Adrenoceptor stimulation typically shifts the voltage-dependent activation of the f-channel toward less negative potentials, thus increasing channel availability at physiologically relevant potentials. That means that the contribution of I_f to the diastolic phase of the action potential increases during β-adrenoceptor stimulation, and may favor the appearance of spontaneous action potentials and arrhythmias.

the two important regulatory systems, the type 1 β-adrenoceptor kinase (βARK1) and the inhibitory G protein (Gi) (Bristow et al, 1986; Neumann et al, 1988; Ungerer et al, 1993). The downregulation of β-adrenoceptor density is specifically limited to the $β_1$-adrenoceptor subtype, the density of $β_2$-adrenoceptor subtype remaining unchanged (Bristow et al, 1986). The pacemaker channel is typically modulated by cyclic nucleotides. This is true for both the native channel (DiFrancesco and Tortora, 1991) and channel isoforms re-expressed in heterologous cell lines (Ludwig et al, 1999a; Moroni et al, 2000). Although several receptors are linked to the cyclic adenosine monophosphate (cAMP) pathway, via either stimulatory or inhibitory G proteins, the β-adrenoceptor pathway is of utmost pathophysiological importance in ventricular myocytes. β-Adrenoceptor stimulation with isoproterenol increases I_f amplitude in both human (Figure 4, left panel) and rat ventricular myocytes (Figure 4, right panel). In both cases, currents were elicited by a double-pulse protocol, during which the cell was hyperpolarized first to −80 mV, to activate half of the current, and then to −120 mV, to activate I_f completely. β-Adrenoceptor stimulation increased the amount of current recorded during the step to −80 mV, and decreased the tail current measured at −120 mV: this behavior is typically attributable to a positive shift in the activation curve of I_f.

Thus, the action of catecholamines on the pacemaker current in ventricular myocytes resembles qualitatively that reported in sinoatrial node myocytes (DiFrancesco, 1993). Further studies have demonstrated that the effect mediated by the $β_1$-adrenoceptor subtype is, however, much greater than that of the $β_2$-adrenoceptor subtype. Some of these differences can be explained by the simultaneous coupling of $β_2$-adrenoceptor to both stimulatory and inhibitory pertussis-toxin–sensitive G proteins; this latter pathway, which is not activated by the $β_1$-adrenoceptor subtype, might limit the effects mediated by the activation of the "primary" pathway, involving the stimulatory G proteins and the cAMP cascade (Xiao et al, 1995). Results obtained in hypertrophied rat myocytes (Cerbai et al, 1999a) and failing human myocytes (Sartiani et al, 1999) further support this view: in fact, the effect of β_2-adrenoceptor stimulation on I_f was significantly increased in cells preincubated with pertussis toxin. However, the stimulation of the β_1-adrenoceptor subtype causes a significantly greater effect on I_f than the β_2-adrenoceptor subtype. Even after pertussis toxin treatment, the shift in the I_f activation curve observed with β_2-adrenoceptor stimulation never reached the amplitude of that caused by β_1-adrenoceptor stimulation. Thus, it may be speculated that the intrinsic activity of β_2-adrenoceptor stimulation on I_f is less effective than that of β_1-adrenoceptor stimulation, not only because the β_2-adrenoceptor subtype is simultaneously coupled to a stimulatory and a pertussis toxin-sensitive inhibitory G protein, but also because other postreceptor mechanisms (e.g., cAMP compartmentation) are operative. Notwithstanding the molecular mechanism(s) underlying these differences, an increase in the inhibitory tone due to Gi activity (Neumann et al, 1988) and the relative upregulation of β_2-adrenoceptors in myocardial hypertrophy and failure (Bristow et al, 1986; Castellano and Bohm, 1997) may be seen as important adaptive changes counteracting the increased arrhythmogenic hazard present in cardiac hypertrophy and failure (i.e., the overexpression of the pacemaker current I_f).

I_f IN HUMAN VENTRICULAR MYOCYTES

In myocytes isolated from human hearts explanted for terminal heart failure due to ischemic cardiomyopathy, I_f was activated in the range of the physiological potentials of those ventricular myocytes (Cerbai et al, 1997), thus supporting the hypothesis of a functional role in the arrhythmogenesis of the failing heart. However, Hoppe et al (1998), while confirming the presence of I_f in human ventricular myocytes, found that myocytes from patients with terminal heart failure had only a trend (not statistically significant) toward increased I_f density compared with myocytes from nonfailing control hearts. They found no statistically significant difference among average current densities measured in 50 myocytes from 23 patients with dilated cardiomyopathy and 30 myocytes from 11 patients with ischemic cardiomyopathy (Hoppe et al, 1998). The experiments were, in most cases, performed at 22°C. The findings were the same when current densities were compared at 22°C and 37°C separately.

To clarify these points, the electrophysiological properties of myocytes from four human hearts that were not used for transplantation for technical reasons (control) were studied; furthermore, I_f was measured in many other hearts explanted for ischemic and idiopathic dilated cardiomyopathy. To gain insight into the possible pathophysiological role of I_f, its densities and properties in these different groups were compared (Cerbai et al, 2001). It was reasoned that if I_f is not a bystander but rather a relevant phenomenon, one should expect, as previously observed in the animal model of hypertrophy and failure (Cerbai et al, 1994b; Cerbai et al, 1996; Cerbai et al, 1995; Cerbai et al, 1997), a greater density in diseased hearts compared with that in normal hearts and a modulation by disease, that is, differences in I_f properties as a function of the etiology of heart failure.

Whole-cell membrane capacitance (C_m) was measured in all the myocytes used to assess the presence and amplitude of I_f. C_m was 218 ± 15 pF in 47 control myocytes; C_m was significantly larger only in myocytes ($n=49$) from dilated cardiomyopathy hearts (333 ± 24 pF), while in those from ischemic cardiomyopathy ($n=39$) the value was 271 ± 24 pF, not statistically different from the control. I_f was recorded in all cells investigated from both ischemic cardiomyopathy and dilated cardiomyopathy hearts. However, I_f could be recorded in 75% of myocytes from normal hearts. In these cells, the mean amplitude measured at -120 mV was significantly lower than in ischemic cardiomyopathy, and dilated cardiomyopathy myocytes. When I_f amplitude was normalized to C_m, the resulting current density was significantly larger in myocytes from ischemic cardiomyopathy (2.0 ± 0.2 pA/pF) compared with control (1.0 ± 0.1 pA/pF) or dilated cardiomyopathy hearts (1.2 ± 0.1 pA/pF). Typical action potentials and I_f recordings from control, ischemic cardiomyopathy, and dilated cardiomyopathy myocytes are shown in Figure 5.

The action potential duration is clearly prolonged in the failing myocytes compared with control (Cerbai et al, 1999c). From a holding potential of -40 mV, hyperpolarizing steps in 10 mV increments

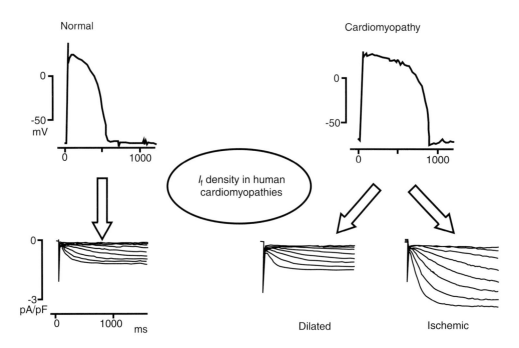

Figure 5 Electrophysiological alterations in the failing human heart. A prolongation of action potential duration (top recordings) and the appearance of the pacemaker current. I_f (bottom traces) are consistently recorded in failing human myocytes. Data obtained in myocytes from nondiseased donor hearts (normal) or diseased explanted hearts (failing) suggest that the functional expression of I_f depends on the etiology of heart failure. In fact, myocytes isolated from the hearts of patients undergoing transplantation for terminal heart failure due to ischemic cardiomyopathy exhibit a significantly greater I_f density than myocytes isolated from patients with idiopathic dilated cardiomyopathy or from normal donor hearts (bottom traces).

elicited a time-dependent inward current that typically increased with hyperpolarization to more negative potentials. Voltage of half maximal activation was significantly shifted to more positive values from a control value of -80.6 ± 1.8 mV to -71.0 ± 1.9 mV in ischemic cardiomyopathy and -74.0 ± 1.3 mV in dilated cardiomyopathy, suggesting that I_f might play a more important functional—and possibly arrhythmogenic—role in ventricular cells from the ischemic myocardium.

CONCLUSIONS

I_f, a current typically found in pacemaker cells, is overexpressed in left ventricular myocytes isolated from severely hypertrophied or failing rat hearts. Many factors (including aging, degree of myocardial hypertrophy, stimulation of β-adrenoceptors) can influence its functional expression. Since hypertrophy induces re-expression of genes encoding fetal proteins, I_f occurrence in this setting may be due to upregulation of a channel present during fetal life. In ventricular myocytes from newborn rats, I_f occurrence and density are maximal at one to two days after birth and progressively decrease during development: at one month, a minority of myocytes expresses I_f, which, when present, has a small amplitude. I_f is also consistently present in human ventricular myocytes isolated from explanted failing hearts, where its expression is influenced by the etiology of the disease. In fact, I_f is present in all cells isolated from patients with terminal heart failure due to ischemic or dilated cardiomyopathy and in 75% of cells from control donor hearts. Moreover, I_f density is significantly higher in ischemic than in either dilated or control human ventricular myocytes. However, membrane capacitance, an index of cell size and hypertrophy, is significantly higher in myocytes from dilated hearts than from ischemic or control hearts. Thus, it appears that I_f is overexpressed in ventricular myocytes isolated from human failing hearts; its expression seems to depend on the etiology of the disease rather than on the degree of cellular hypertrophy. I_f may represent a relevant arrhythmogenic trigger in the failing heart.

For example, the overexpression of the depolarizing current I_f may increase (particularly under the influence of β-adrenoceptor stimulation) the likelihood that a subthreshold delayed after depolarization, a frequent event in hypertrophied or failing myocyte, may reach the threshold and trigger an arrhythmia in a heart where the substrate for reentry is certainly present. Obviously, it must be kept in mind that many other cellular electrophysiological changes occur in the hypertrophied and failing heart and all may contribute to the phenomenon of electrophysiological remodeling.

ACKNOWLEDGMENTS

We warmly thank Prof Guido Sani, Dr Massimo Maccherini, and all the people involved in the heart transplantation program for their invaluable and enthusiastic collaboration. The original work presented here was supported by grants from MURST and Telethon.

CHAPTER 4

MOLECULAR STRUCTURE AND FUNCTIONAL EXPRESSION OF I_f CHANNELS FROM HEART AND CENTRAL NERVOUS SYSTEM

MARTIN BIEL

INTRODUCTION

The autonomous beating of the heart is controlled by specialized pacemaker cells in the sinoatrial (SA) node that generate spontaneous, rhythmic electrical impulses in the absence of any external input (DiFrancesco, 1993). In the brain, a number of different regions are also capable of generating spontaneous rhythms. Such rhythmic firing patterns are believed to control important physiological functions, such as the sleep-wake cycle (McCormick and Bal, 1997), respiration (Ramirez and Richter, 1996), and the ability of the brain to bind different sensory inputs into a single percept (Singer and Gray, 1995). The generation of pacemaker potentials relies on a complex interplay between at least four different types of cation channels: T- and L-type Ca^{2+} channels, K^+ channels, and a cation channel, termed I_f (synonymous with I_h and I_q). The I_f channel has also been designated as "pacemaker" channel because it reveals unique features that are believed to be a prerequisite for pacemaker activity (DiFrancesco, 1993; Pape, 1996). First, unlike most voltage-gated channels, which open when the membrane potential becomes depolarized, I_f channels open upon membrane hyperpolarization. Second, I_f channels display only a weak selectivity for K^+ over Na^+; as a result, the reversal potential of these channels lies at around -25 mV, so they carry an inward current at the hyperpolarized potentials where they open. This depolarizing inward current, starting at the end of the repolarization phase of the action potential, drives the membrane potential back towards threshold at which calcium channels activate, thereby maintaining rhythmic firing. Third, cyclic adenosine monophosphate (cAMP) binds to I_f channels and, hence, shifts their voltage dependence of activation to more positive voltages. Thus, in the presence of high cellular cAMP concentrations, I_f channel opening is faster and more complete than at low cAMP levels. It is this cAMP-mediated enhancement of channel activity that accounts for the positive chronotropic effect of β-adrenergic agonists in the heart (DiFrancesco and Tortora, 1991). Conversely, hormones and neurotransmitters that lower the cellular cAMP level inhibit the rate and extent to which I_f channels open after an action potential and, hence, reduce the firing frequency of pacemaker potentials (DiFrancesco et al, 1989). Apart from their key role in cardiac and neuronal pacemaking, I_f channels fulfill diverse functions in cell types that do not develop spontaneous electrical activity. Examples for such "nonpacemaking" functions are the generation of rebound depolarizations in retinal photoreceptors (Fain et al, 1978; Wollmuth and Hille, 1992), the control of synaptic plasticity (Beaumont and Zucker, 2000), and the integration of synaptic inputs (Magee, 1999).

MOLECULAR CLONING OF I_f CHANNELS—THE HCN GENE FAMILY

Several cDNAs encoding I_f channels have been isolated by molecular cloning (Gauss et al, 1998; Ludwig et al, 1998; Santoro et al, 1997, 1998; for a complete list of cloned channels, see Kaupp and Seifert, 2001). With regard to their dual mode of activation, the channels were termed hyperpolarization-activated and cyclic nucleotide-gated cation (HCN) channels. In vertebrates, the HCN channel family comprises four members (HCN1, HCN2, HCN3, and HCN4). HCN channels were also cloned from some invertebrates, but are not represented in the genome of the nematode *C elegans* (Littleton and Ganetzky, 2000). Hydropathicity analysis and sequence comparisons classify HCN channels as members of the superfamily of voltage-gated cation channels (Figure 1a,b). The channels are distantly related (about 20–25% overall sequence identity) to eag (ether-a-go-go) K^+ channels (Warmke and Ganetzky, 1994) and to the cyclic nucleotide-gated (CNG) channel class (Biel et al, 1999). HCN channels contain six membrane-spanning helices (S1 to S6), including a positively charged voltage-sensing S4 segment and an ion-conducting pore between S5 and S6. In the C-terminus, the channels carry a cyclic nucleotide-binding domain (CNBD), which is highly conserved in a variety of other cyclic nucleotide-binding proteins including cAMP- and cyclic guanosine monophosphate (cGMP)–activated protein kinases (Pfeifer et al, 1999), cAMP-binding guanine nucleotide exchange factors (GEFs) (Kawasaki et al, 1998; de Rooij et al, 1998), and CNG channels (Biel et al, 1999). The core region of the channels spanning from S1 to the C-terminus of the CNBD is highly conserved within the HCN channel family (80–90% sequence identity; Figure 1b). In contrast, N- and C-termini of the channels vary considerably in their length and share only modest sequence homology. Analogous to other members of the superfamily of voltage-gated cation channels, HCN channels probably assemble to tetrameric complexes. Heterologously expressed HCN channels exhibit the hallmark properties of native I_f, that is, activation upon membrane hyperpolarization, conduction of Na^+ and K^+, enhancement by cyclic nucleotides, and blockage by extracellular Cs^+ (Ishii et al, 1999; Ludwig et al, 1998, 1999b; Moosmang et al, 2001; Santoro et al, 1998; Seifert et al, 1999). While this finding suggests that I_f channels are homomeric complexes, there is also preliminary evidence that, at least in Xenopus oocytes, HCN1 and HCN2 can associate to form a heteromeric channel with novel properties (Ulens and Tytgat, 2001). Studies with specific antibodies will be necessary to determine the subunit composition and the stoichiometry of the channels *in vivo*. It also remains to be determined whether native I_f channels like Ca^{2+} or K^+ channels contain auxilliary subunits that are associated with the principal pore-forming subunits.

STRUCTURAL DETERMINANTS OF HCN CHANNEL FUNCTION

Channel activation by voltage and cyclic nucleotides

One of the most remarkable features of HCN channels is their complex mechanism of activation. HCN channels belong to the class of voltage-gated channels because their activation obligatorily requires membrane hyperpolarization. However, the channels are also ligand-gated because cyclic nucleotides enhance channel activity by altering the voltage dependence of channel activation. This dual activation mode is mirrored in the primary sequence of HCN channels, which contains both a positively charged voltage sensor (S4 segment) and a CNBD. There are two alternative hypotheses to explain the gating of HCN channels. In the first model, which is derived from models of HERG (human ether-a-go-go-related gene) K^+ channel gating (Smith et al, 1996), opening is due to recovery of channels from an inactivated state. Such a "recovery from inactivation" model is supported by site-directed mutagenesis experiments showing that neutralization of positively charged residues in the S4 of HCN2 does not alter the general characteristics of the channel but shifts the voltage dependence of channel activation to even more hyperpolarized voltages (Chen et al, 2000; Vaca et al, 2000). A competing hypothesis is that hyperpolarization-dependent channel opening represents activation from a normal closed state (Zei and Aldrich, 1998). This model suggests that in both depolarization- and hyperpolarization-activated channels, the movement of S4 is coupled to the channel gate but with the opposite polarity, that is, the activation gate is closed when the S4 is in its outermost configuration at positive voltages in HCN channels but open in other channels. In order to determine which hypothesis is correct, it will be necessary in the future to measure gating currents of HCN channels.

HCN channels activate with a characteristic sigmoidal time course. The current (with the exception of an initial lag phase) is usually fitted by either mono- or biexponential functions (Pape, 1996). The time constants of activation (τ) are strongly voltage-dependent becoming increasingly larger the more the plasma membrane is depolarized. The different HCN channels display different kinetics (Table 1). HCN1 is the fastest channel (τ at -140 mV = 30 ms) followed by HCN2, HCN3, and HCN4. HCN4 is by far the slowest channel displaying activation constants ranging between a few hundred milliseconds at strongly hyperpolarized voltages (-140 mV) up to several seconds at normal resting potential (-70 mV).

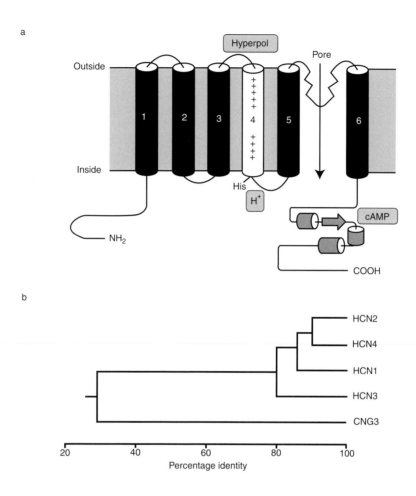

Figure 1 a: Model of the transmembrane structure of HCN channels. The six transmembrane segments S1–S6 are numbered 1–6. The ion-conducting pore is localized between S5 and S6. The positively charged S4 segment that confers channel gating upon hyperpolarization and the carboxy terminal cyclic nucleotide-binding domain that confers channel activation by cAMP are indicated. The histidine residue (His321) at the interface between S4 and the S4–S5 linker, which is a major determinant of pH sensitivity, is highlighted. b: Phylogenetic tree of the HCN channel family. The tree was calculated by comparison of the corresponding regions from segment S1 to the end of the cyclic nucleotide-binding domain. c: Comparison of the pore region of HCN1-4 with that of the human potassium channel Kv1.1 (Browne et al, 1994) and the bovine CNG3 channel (Biel et al, 1994). SF, selectivity filter (Doyle et al, 1998). The relative permeability ratio P_{Na}/P_K is given for the respective channels. cAMP, cyclic adenosine monophosphate.

TABLE 1 Functional properties and tissue distribution of HCN channels.

	HCN1	HCN2	HCN3	HCN4
Human gene locus	nd	19p13.3	nd	15q24-q25
$V_{0.5}$ (whole cell mode) [mV]	−94	−99	−96	−100
Activation constant (τ) at −140 mV [ms]	30	184	265	461
P_{Na}/P_K	0.25	0.24	nd	0.22
cAMP-induced shift of $V_{0.5}$ [mV]	+2–4	+15	nd	+15
Distribution of HCN channel mRNA in mouse tissues				
Heart				
Ventricular myocytes	−	++	−	+
Atrial myocytes	−	+/++	−	+
SA node	−/+	+/++	−	+++
Retina				
Photoreceptors	+++	−	−	−
Inner nuclear layer	++	+	++	−
Ganglion cells	++	+	++	−
Dorsal root ganglia	+++	++	−	−
Brain				
Neocortex	+++	++	+/−	+/−
Hippocampus CA1-3	+/+++	++	+/−	+
Thalamus	+/−	+++	+/−	++
Brainstem	−	+++	+/−	+/−

Electrophysiological data for the heterologously expressed murine HCN1–3 and the human HCN4 channel were compiled from Ludwig et al (1999b) and Moosmang et al (2001). The tissue distribution data are based on in situ hybridizations and were taken from Moosmang et al (1999, 2001). +++, strong; ++, moderate; +, low; +/−, very low, −, no expression, nd, not determined.

The effect of cyclic nucleotides on HCN channel activity is complex, comprising a shift of the activation curve towards more positive membrane potentials (Table 1) and an acceleration of the activation kinetics. Cyclic nucleotides regulate HCN channel activity independently of a protein kinase–mediated modification by directly binding to a CNBD in the C-terminus of the protein (DiFrancesco and Tortora, 1991; Gauss et al, 1998; Ludwig et al, 1998). As mentioned above, the CNBD of HCN channels is homologous to CNBDs found in a number of other cyclic nucleotide–binding proteins. The highest degree of sequence identity (about 45%) is seen for the CNBD of the CNG channels. Despite this close structural relationship, HCN channels reveal an approximately 10-fold higher affinity for cAMP than for cGMP (K_a = 0.5 µM for cAMP and 6 µM for cGMP in the expressed murine HCN2 channel; Ludwig et al, 1998), whereas most CNG channels strongly select cGMP over cAMP (Biel et al, 1999; Zagotta and Siegelbaum, 1996). The molecular determinants of the cAMP specificity of HCN channels have not been identified so far; however, site-directed mutagenesis in CNG channels suggests that the C-terminus of the CNBD (the so-called αC-helix) might play a major role in controlling cyclic nucleotide preference. Within the αC helix of CNG channels a negatively charged amino acid (D604 in the CNG1 channel) confers selectivity for cGMP over cAMP (Varnum et al, 1995). Replacement of D604 by neutral amino acids results in CNG channels that no longer select cGMP over cAMP. It will be interesting to see whether the isoleucine that is present in the αC-helix of HCN channels at the position corresponding to D604 is an important control element for the cAMP preference of HCN channels.

In contrast to other HCN channels, HCN1 is only marginally affected by cyclic nucleotides, if at all (Figure 2; see also Santoro et al, 1998; Ulens and Tytgat, 2001). It is difficult to decide whether the observed shift of the activation curve of about 2–4 mV is of physiological relevance. In any case, the low degree of cyclic nucleotide modulation in HCN1 is rather unexpected given the high percentage of

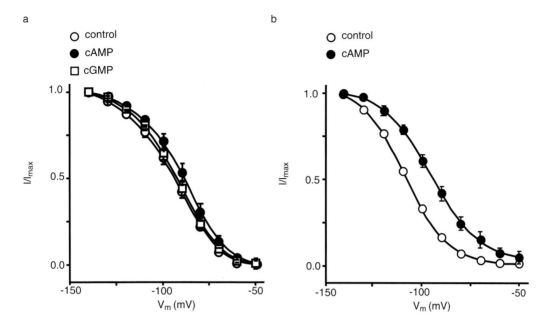

Figure 2a: Voltage-dependence of murine HCN1 channel activation measured in whole-cell current mode under control conditions or after pipette perfusion with either 1 mM cAMP or cGMP for at least one minute. Activation curves were constructed using tail current analysis as follows: the cells were clamped from a holding potential of −40 mV to test potential ranging from −50 mV to −140 mV in 10 mV increments for 200 ms, followed by a step to −140 mV. Tail currents were measured immediately after the step to −140 mV. The solid lines represent fits of the data to the Boltzmann function. The $V_{0.5}$ as deduced from the fitting was not significantly different between control (−94 mV), cAMP (−90 mV), and cGMP (−93 mV). b: Activation curves of human HCN4 measured under control conditions and after perfusion with 1 mM cAMP. The pulse protocol was as described in Figure 2a with the exception that the pulse duration was 10 s. $V_{0.5}$ deduced from Boltzmann fits was −108 mV for control and −93 mV in the presence of cAMP. cAMP, cyclic adenosine monophosphate; cGMP, cyclic guanosine monophosphate.

sequence conservation (over 90%) between the CNBD of HCN1 and those of HCN2 or HCN4. Thus, it is not very likely that the loss of cAMP modulation in HCN1 results from the inability of the channel to bind cyclic nucleotides. Rather, a functional defect in the conformational step that couples cyclic nucleotide binding to channel gating may underlie the differences in cyclic nucleotide sensitivity. In CNG channels, domains that are localized outside of the CNBD, such as the so-called C-linker (Zong et al, 1998) or the cytoplasmic N-terminus (Goulding et al, 1994), control channel activation. It is thus tempting to speculate that these domains may also determine the extent by which cyclic nucleotides modulate HCN channel activity.

ION SELECTIVITY

HCN channels are mixed cation channels conducting both Na^+ and K^+ ions with a relative permeability ratio P_{Na}/P_K of about 0.2–0.25 (Gauss et al, 1998; Ho et al, 1994; Ludwig et al, 1998; Santoro et al, 1998). Due to this particular ion selectivity, HCN currents, at physiological ionic conditions, reverse at around −25 mV. As a consequence, the channels carry depolarizing inward Na^+ currents at resting potential. While HCN channels pass both K^+ and Na^+, they are not nonselective. HCN channels are almost impermeable to Li^+ and are even blocked by millimolar concentrations of Cs^+. Similarly, divalents and anions do not pass through the channels. Although HCN channels conduct mainly Na^+ under physiological conditions, the primary sequence of the HCN pore region is clearly related to that of highly selective

K⁺ channels, while the sequence homology to pores of nonselective CNG channels or sodium channels is much weaker (Figure 1c). In contrast to the latter channels, both K⁺ and HCN channels contain a glycine-tyrosine-glycine motif in the pore. In tetrameric K⁺ channels, four copies of this sequence form the narrowest part of the pore providing the selectivity filter for K⁺ ions (Doyle et al, 1998; Heginbotham et al, 1994). The presence of the GYG sequence in HCN channels indicates that this motif alone is not sufficient to induce selectivity for K⁺. By affecting the spatial coordination of the GYG sequences in the tetrameric channel complex, other channel domains could control the structural rigidity of the pore and, hence, determine whether only K⁺ or also other monovalents are allowed to permeate. In this context, it is notable that K⁺ is not only a permeating cation but also a regulator of Na⁺ permeation (Frace et al, 1992a; Ludwig et al, 1998; Wollmuth and Hille, 1992). The P_{Na}/P_K ratio and the amplitude of the HCN current critically depend on the extracellular K⁺ concentration. In the absence of extracellular K⁺, the inward Na⁺ current is abolished. The interdependence of K⁺ and Na⁺ permeation supports the idea that HCN channels like CNG and Ca²⁺ channels are multi-ion pores possessing at least two cation binding sites with different affinities for Na⁺ and K⁺, respectively. Although HCN channels conduct cationic currents, extracellular Cl⁻ is needed for channel activity (Frace et al, 1992b; Santoro et al, 1998). Substitution of Cl⁻ by larger anions such as isothionate or gluconate results in a pronounced reduction of the current amplitude. This finding suggests that the pore of HCN channels contains an extracellular binding site for Cl⁻, which may be related to the presence of up to three positively charged residues in this region (Figure 1c).

CHANNEL MODULATION

A physiologically important property of I_f channels is their ability to be regulated by neurotransmitters and metabolic stimuli (Pape, 1996). In most cases, the regulation relies on a shift of the voltage-dependence of channel activation to either positive or negative direction. As discussed above, cAMP shifts the HCN channel activation curve to more positive membrane potentials. Thus, channel activity is enhanced by neurotransmitters like norepinephrine which activate adenylyl cyclase, whereas it is decreased by substances like acetylcholine which inhibit cAMP synthesis. While there is no longer any doubt that cAMP modulates HCN channels by directly binding to the channel, it is still possible that cAMP could exert some additional effect on HCN channels via cAMP-dependent protein kinase (PKA)-mediated phosphorylation (Chang et al, 1991). There is a highly conserved serine residue in the CNBD of HCN channels (Ser641 in murine HCN2), which could serve as a target for PKA phosphorylation. It was also reported that neurotransmitters regulate I_f in a membrane delimited pathway by activating G proteins (Yatani et al, 1990). However, this hypothesis has not yet been substantiated by further experiments (see also Pape, 1996).

Similarly, the physiological relevance of Ca²⁺- and cGMP-dependent upregulation of HCN channel activity is still a matter of controversy (discussed in Pape, 1996). A study with thalamocortical neurons indicates that the activity of these neurons can be controlled by nitric oxide via stimulation of cGMP synthesis and subsequent activation of I_f (Pape and Mager, 1992). This finding suggests that cGMP may be an important cellular regulator of the channels, at least in neurons. Like cAMP, cyclic GMP could also act indirectly on the channels, for example, by activating cGMP-dependent protein kinases or by inhibiting phosphodiesterases and, thereby, increasing the cAMP level.

There is recent evidence that I_f channels are regulated by changes in intracellular pH (Munsch and Pape, 1999). Protons shift the voltage-dependence of channel activation to more hyperpolarizing voltages and slow down the speed of activation. Thus, at acidic pH, channel activity will be low, whereas it is enhanced under alkaline conditions. The modulation of HCN channels by internal pH could be involved in the control of a variety of physiological processes, including thalamic oscillations, respiratory frequency, and sperm motility. Inhibition of HCN channel activity by acidosis could also be important under pathological conditions, such as heart failure and myocardial infarction. Site-directed mutagenesis has been used to identify a protonable histidine residue in murine HCN2 (His321; Figure 1a), which is a major determinant of pH sensitivity (Zong et al, 2001). The residue is localized at the boundary between the voltage-sensing S4 segment and the cytoplasmic S4–S5 linker. This localization is very consistent with a possible role of the residue in modulating channel gating. Because the identified histidine residue is conserved in all four vertebrate HCN channel isoforms, regulation by intracellular pH is likely to constitute a general feature of both cardiac and neuronal I_f channels.

TISSUE EXPRESSION OF HCN CHANNELS

Expression in heart

In situ hybridization, reverse transcriptase-polymerase chain reaction (RT-PCR), and Northern blot analysis identified three HCN channel types (HCN1, HCN2, and HCN4) in the heart (Ishii et al, 1999; Ludwig et al, 1998, 1999b; Shi et al, 1999). In murine SA node pacemaker cells, HCN4 is by far the predominant HCN channel type expressed (Table 1). In addition to HCN4, murine SA node contains low levels of HCN2 (about 10-fold less than HCN4) and trace amounts of HCN1. HCN4 was also identified as the major HCN channel in the SA node of rabbit heart. Unlike the mouse SA node cells, rabbit pacemaker cells contain moderate levels of HCN1 (about a quarter of the HCN4 expression level) but almost completely lack HCN2. HCN3 was not detected in SA node or any other region of the heart. So far, no data on the expression of HCN channels in human SA node are available. HCN channels are also present in heart muscle, in which HCN2 is the major isoform. In addition, minor amounts of HCN4 have been found in human and mouse, but not in rabbit, cardiomyocytes.

The presence of HCN channels in diverse types of heart cells is consistent with reports describing I_f currents in ventricular (Hoppe et al, 1998; Yu et al, 1995) and atrial myocytes (Thuringer et al, 1992) as well as in conduction tissues (DiFrancesco, 1993). The I_f current from ventricular myocytes differs significantly from that of SA node cells in the voltage dependence of activation. Half-maximal activation potentials ($V_{0.5}$) determined for I_f in ventricular myocytes range from −95 to −135 mV, whereas I_f in SA node cells activates at more positive potentials with $V_{0.5}$ ranging from −65 to −90 mV. The reason for the differing $V_{0.5}$ values is unknown. However, $V_{0.5}$ values as well as activation constants strongly depend on experimental conditions, such as the length of the hyperpolarizing activation pulse, ionic milieu, cAMP concentration, pH value, temperature, and electrophysiological configuration (whole-cell versus excised patch mode). This variability could well explain why, even for the same channel, differences in $V_{0.5}$ values of 25 to 30 mV have been reported (Ludwig et al, 1999b; Seifert et al, 1999). Thus, as a basis for further interpretations, it will be necessary to measure native and cloned HCN channels under standardized conditions. Differences in $V_{0.5}$ that persist might be attributed to the absence or presence of auxilliary channel subunits, the formation of heteromeric HCN channels, or the action of cellular factors on HCN channels.

EXPRESSION IN NEURONS

Transcripts of all four HCN channels are present in mouse (Moosmang et al, 1999, 2001; Santoro et al, 2000) and rat (Monteggia et al, 2000) brain. The expression levels and the regional distribution of the HCN channel mRNAs vary profoundly between the respective channel types. HCN2 is the most abundant neuronal channel and is found almost ubiquitously in the brain. In contrast, HCN1 and HCN4 are enriched in specific regions of the brain (Table 1). HCN3 is uniformly expressed throughout the brain, but at very low levels. The expression pattern of the individual HCN channel types in the brain has been summarized in great detail in recent articles (Monteggia et al, 2000; Moosmang et al, 1999; Santoro et al, 2000) and, therefore, will not be further discussed in this review.

Historically, the I_f current was discovered for the first time in rod photoreceptors (Fain et al, 1978). In these cells, I_f functions as a feedback current that produces rebound depolarizations when the cell becomes hyperpolarized in response to bright light. In situ hybridizations identified high levels of HCN1 transcripts in photoreceptors of the murine retina, whereas HCN2–4 were not found in these cells

(Table 1). HCN1 is also found together with HCN2 and HCN3 in ganglion cells and the inner nuclear layer of the retina, which contains the cell bodies of bipolar, amacrine, Müller glial, and horizontal cells. In contrast, transcripts for HCN4 were not detected in murine retina. The presence of HCN1, HCN2, and HCN3 channels in various retinal cell types indicates that these channels fulfill diverse functions in the neural circuitry that confers vision.

I_f channels have also been characterized in peripheral neurons (for a review, see Pape, 1996). For example, dorsal root ganglion (DRG) neurons, which are committed to the transmission of proprioceptive, nociceptive, and thermal information, express HCN1 and HCN2 channels (Moosmang et al, 2001). The identification of these channels agrees well with the characterization of I_f currents in DRG neurons (Mayer and Westbrook, 1983) and suggests that HCN channels may have a general function in the transmission of sensory information in the body.

CONCLUSION

The molecular cloning of the HCN gene family has provided the basis to achieve a deeper understanding of I_f channels. A number of important questions can now be addressed. What is the molecular basis of the dual activation by hyperpolarization and cyclic nucleotides? Which channel domains determine the unique ion selectivity? What is the subunit composition of native HCN channels? Which cellular factors regulate the channels *in vivo*? Finally, the powerful approaches of mouse genetics will allow the definition of specific functions that each of the four HCN channels fulfills in the body. Furthermore, it should now be possible to determine whether mutations in pacemaker channel genes may underlie genetic diseases, such as cardiac arrhythmia, certain types of seizures, or other neurological disorders.

ACKNOWLEDGMENT

This work was supported by the Deutsche Forschungsgemeinschaft.

CHAPTER 5

CHANGES IN HEART RATE AND ACTIVATION PATHWAY AND THEIR ROLE IN MODIFYING CARDIAC REPOLARIZATION

MICHAEL R. ROSEN, ALEXEI PLOTNIKOV, RAVIL GAINULLIN, PARAG CHANDRA, BENGT HERWEG, AND PETER DANILO JR

INTRODUCTION

The evolution of the heart from a tubular structure to the four-chambered organ of adult mammals is accompanied by the localization of sinus node impulse initiation to a discrete region in the right atrium and the development of a specialized conduction system that carries the cardiac impulse from the sinus node to the working myocardium of the atria and ventricles. There is a complex relationship between the site of impulse initiation in the heart—whether sinus node or ectopic pacemaker—the pathways via which cardiac excitation proceeds, and the process of repolarization. This relationship is the subject to be discussed here.

Impulse initiation in the sinus node largely derives from the pacemaker current I_f, an inward current carried by sodium ions that is activated on hyperpolarization of the cell membrane (DiFrancesco, 1985, 1991). Although the sinus node is the primary source of impulse initiation, most cardiac myocytes also have I_f. However, in cells outside the sinus node, I_f activates at potentials quite negative to those of the node. These potentials are out of the physiologic range of membrane potentials of atrial and ventricular muscle (Robinson et al, 1997; Yu et al, 1993). Interestingly, in certain pathologic states (e.g., hypertension, congestive failure), the activation threshold of I_f in myocardium becomes more positive (Cerbai et al, 1994b) such that there is at least a theoretical basis for expecting that it might give rise to competing rhythms in the heart.

There are several situations in which sites of impulse initiation in the heart may be altered. There may be a change in pacemaker location, involving the normal pacemaker current; abnormal automatic rhythms may be initiated by depolarized cardiac fibers; or triggered activity may occur as a result of early or delayed afterdepolarizations (see Wit and Rosen, 1986, for a review). The implantation of electrical pacemakers provides another means whereby the site of origin of the cardiac impulse is altered. In any of the above settings, the pathway of activation is highly likely to change. It may also change in the setting of reentrant rhythms (Janse and Wit, 1989).

Hence, in a variety of circumstances, activation of the heart is altered. Not long ago, the work of Mauricio Rosenbaum and associates on cardiac memory (Rosenbaum et al, 1982, 1983) inspired us (del Balzo and Rosen, 1992; Rosen et al, 1998) and others (Costard-Jäckle et al, 1989; Katz, 1992) to consider the impact of altering the activation pathway on the repolarization of the heart. In this paper, we review data obtained using pacing of the atria or the ventricles to understand the impact of altered activation on repolarization. Given that the site of pacing is localized, the results obtained can be thought of as surrogates for the effects on activation of a focal site of impulse initiation or reentry.

METHODS

Studies were conducted in accordance with institutional rules for animal experimentation.

STUDIES OF VENTRICLE

Mongrel dogs weighing 24–26 kg were anesthetized with thiopental sodium (17 mg/kg intravenously), and ventilated with isoflurane (1.5%–2%) and O_2 (2 L/min). Morphine sulfate (0.15 mg/kg) was injected epidurally for postoperative analgesia. Using sterile techniques, a unipolar pacing lead (Medtronic model 6917) was attached to the anteroseptal or posterolateral left ventricular (LV) epicardium. The lead was connected to a programmable pacemaker (MINIX 8340, Medtronic), placed in a subcutaneous pocket. Platinum bipolar electrodes were also sewn onto the epicardium of the left atrial appendage.

Experiments were performed on conscious animals resting quietly on the right side. A pseudo-orthogonal 3-lead ECG (I, aVF, V_{10}) and the epicardial electrogram recordings were acquired at a 1000 Hz sampling rate using Ponemah software (Gould Instrument Systems, Inc) and the Dr Vetter PC-EKG program (Shvilkin et al, 1998; Plotnikov et al, 2001). Frontal plane vector images were plotted with the Dr Vetter PC-EKG program.

Three to five consecutive cycles of the three pseudo-orthogonal ECG leads were averaged for each experimental time point, and the first derivative of the QRST complex was plotted. Cardiac memory was quantified as a function of amplitude and angle changes of the T wave vector and expressed as displacement (in mV) between frontal plane T vector peaks during atrial pacing at baseline and after memory induction. To test whether frontal plane recordings gave the same information as those from XY and Z planes, we made simultaneous frontal plane (Dr Vetter PC-EKG system) and XYZ loop recordings (MIDA 1000, Ortivus Medical Systems, Sweden) in five dogs over 21 days. Vector quantification was identical in both systems (Plotnikov et al, 2001).

STUDIES OF ATRIUM

A right intercostal thoracotomy was performed and bipolar Medtronic electrodes (model 5058) were attached epicardially to the left atrial (LA) appendage (LAA) and right ventricular free wall. Leads were tunneled subcutaneously and connected to a Medtronic 7864B dual-chamber pulse generator implanted in the right posterior thorax. Bipolar electrodes for pacing and recording were attached to the lateral right atrium (RA) and LAA, subcutaneously tunneled to the right posterior thorax, and exteriorized. Complete heart block was produced by injecting 0.1–0.3 mL of 40% formaldehyde into the basal ventricular septum (Herweg et al, 2001).

Immediately after surgery, the pulse generator was programmed into a VDD mode (rate limits 30 and 150 beats per minute, sensed atrioventricular delay 80 ms). This ensured *P*-synchronous ventricular pacing with a normal PR interval during recovery, thus maintaining a sinus-initiated rhythm and avoiding any atrial remodeling secondary to the AV dyssynchrony that characterizes heart block.

In both protocols, dogs were monitored and stabilized for approximately three weeks, at which time recovery was complete, the ECG was stable (i.e., sinus rhythm with ventricular pacing), and the animals were laboratory-trained.

RESULTS

Ventricular pacing protocols

Pacing the ventricles for brief intervals (≤2 h) produces an alteration in activation pathway and, when pacing ceases, an alteration in the T wave such that it tracks the paced QRS complex (Figure 1). It is this phenomenon that Rosenbaum et al (1982) referred to as cardiac memory. The extent of T wave change increases with the number of paced beats and the duration of pacing. Moreover, reinstitution of pacing after a period in sinus rhythm results in an even greater change in the T wave (Figure 2). This is referred to as accumulation. Over approximately 14 days of continuous pacing, the "new" T wave reaches a maximum beyond which additional pacing does not further influence the magnitude of repolarization change but only its persistence after pacing ceases (Figure 3).

The mechanism responsible for this accumulation of changes in repolarization has been detailed in part. It is clear that when the site of impulse initiation is altered, stress/strain relationships on the myocardium are modified (Ricard et al, 1999). Based on the work of Sadoshima et al (1992), in which altered stretch of myocytes in tissue culture increased their synthesis of angiotensin II, we hypothesized

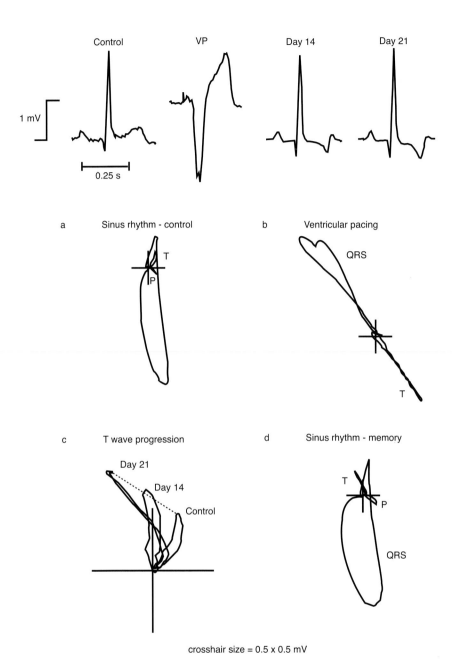

Figure 1 Upper panel. Lead II ECG recorded from a dog in sinus rhythm (control), at the onset of ventricular pacing (VP) at 10% faster than sinus rate and after return to sinus rhythm following 14 and 21 days of ventricular pacing. Note that the QRS complexes are nearly identical to control on days 14 and 21, while the T wave has inverted, consistent with the QRS complex of ventricular pacing. As suggested by Rosenbaum et al (1982), the T wave "remembers" the QRS of the paced rhythm. Panel a shows the P, QRS, and T wave vectors of the animal in sinus rhythm. Panel b shows the paced QRS and T vectors. Panel c is an enlargement of the progression in sinus rhythm T wave vectors from control through days 14 and 21. Note that, as compared with the control, the T wave vector has moved in the direction of the QRS vector in panel b. Panel d shows for comparison purposes with Panel a the P, QRS, and T vectors on day 21. T wave vector displacement (in mV) is measured from the peak of the control T vector to the peak of the day 21 vector (dashed line in panel c). Modified with permission from Shvilkin et al, 1998.

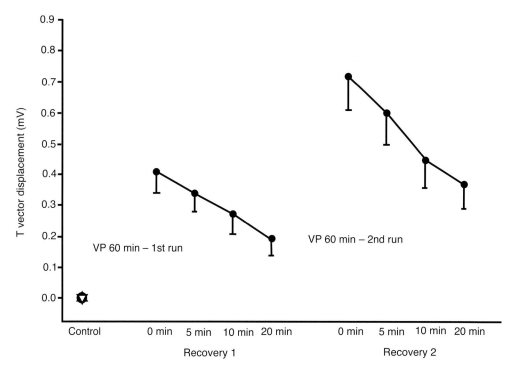

Figure 2 Accumulation of T wave vector changes, as measured in displacement (see Figure 1c for method). Control is expressed as "0". Following 60 min of ventricular pacing at 10% faster than sinus rate, five dogs are paced from the atrium. A displacement of the T wave vector is seen (cardiac memory), which then decays over 20 min. A second run of ventricular pacing for 60 min is instituted. On return to atrial pacing there has been a greater shift in the T vector (referred to as accumulation) and there is a lesser return towards control over the next 20 min. Results expressed as means ± SEM. Modified with permission from Plotnikov et al, 2001.

that when a change in activation site and pathway occurs in the heart, angiotensin II synthesis would increase, thereby initiating a signal transduction pathway that influences repolarization. The likelihood that this is true in the intact animal is seen in experiments in which any of three interventions — an angiotensin II receptor blocker, an angiotensin-converting enzyme inhibitor, or a tissue protease inhibitor — prevented the expression of repolarization changes induced by pacing (Ricard et al, 1999).

The effector pathways distal to the angiotensin II receptor are still not detailed with regard to these repolarization phenomena, but one target, the transient outward current carried by potassium, has been studied in detail (Yu et al, 1999). I_{to} is responsible for phase 1 of myocardial repolarization, and is decreased when chronic pacing is performed to alter the activation pathway. Acute blockade of I_{to} prevents the repolarization changes induced by pacing from occurring at all (del Balzo and Rosen, 1992). The changes in I_{to} relate both to its density and its kinetics. There is a decrease in density by about one third, as well as a shift in activation threshold to more positive voltages and a greater than 10-fold delay in recovery of I_{to} from inactivation (Yu et al, 1999). Moreover, in this setting, *Kv4.3*, the gene responsible for the α subunit of I_{to}, shows an approximately one third reduction in message level (Yu et al, 1999). Interestingly, incubation of epicardial myocytes from control animals with angiotensin II induces changes in I_{to} that are qualitatively and quantitatively identical to those seen with pacing (with comparable changes in current density, activation threshold, and recovery from inactivation) (Yu et al, 2000). This strengthens the argument for a role for angiotensin II in repolarization changes resulting from altered activation.

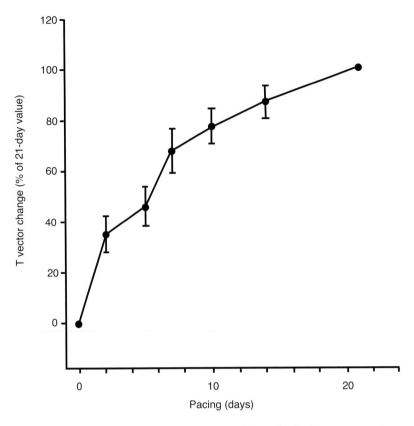

Figure 3 Change in T wave vector displacement (see Fig 1c for method of measurement) over 21 days of ventricular pacing at 10% faster than sinus rate in 16 dogs. Results expressed as % of 21-day value. On the days for which data are reported, ventricular pacing was discontinued for one hour prior to making the T vector measurement in sinus rhythm. Note the accumulation of T wave changes, which reach a peak between days 14 and 21. Although not shown, return to control takes weeks to months (Shvilkin et al, 1998). Results expressed as means ± SEM. Modified with permission from Shvilkin et al, 1998.

The alteration in I_{to} function is accompanied by a change in the transmural gradient for repolarization (Shvilkin et al, 1998). Specifically, action potentials in the epicardium and endocardium prolong, while those in mid-myocardium remain relatively unchanged (Figure 4). Given that I_{to} is not present in endocardium, it is likely that channels other than I_{to} are involved in the induction of the T wave changes: these are being studied at present.

In summary, then, any event that alters the site and/or pathway of ventricular activation can be expected to predictably and consistently modify the repolarization of the ventricle via transduction mechanisms currently under investigation.

ATRIAL PACING PROTOCOLS

The study of repolarization in the atrium is facilitated if we can visualize the Ta waves. For this reason, animals in complete heart block were studied via AV-sequential pacing (Herweg et al, 2001). In this way, the PR interval could be sufficiently prolonged to permit Ta waves to be visualized (Figure 4). In contrast to the T waves of the ventricles, Ta wave changes are often too subtle to be readily quantified from standard ECG leads. We have found it most convenient to consider them in X, Y, and Z projections, after which an atrial gradient (AG) is calculated as follows:

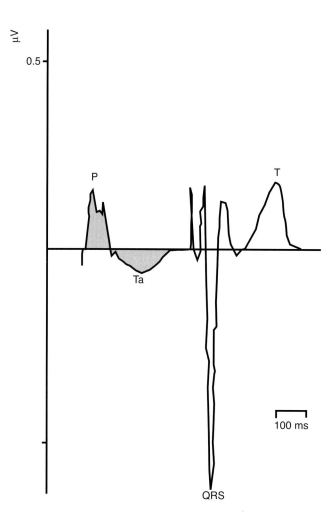

Figure 4 Signal-averaged P and Ta waves in orthogonal lead X during atrioventricular sequential pacing. Complete atrioventricular block allowed sufficient atrioventricular interval prolongation to reveal the entire Ta wave. Modified with permission from Herweg et al, 2001.

$$\text{Spatial AG} = \sqrt{(\text{IPTa}_x)^2 + (\text{IPTa}_y)^2 + (\text{IPTa}_z)^2}$$

Using the ventricle as a model (Rosenbaum et al, 1982; Hayashi et al, 1976a,b), the area of the primary Ta wave should equal the PTa voltage-time integral in X, Y, and Z leads (Herweg et al, 2001). PTa voltage-time integrals and spatial atrial gradient have been considered to measure repolarization independently of activation sequence (Hayashi et al, 1976a,b; Wilson et al, 1934). However, ventricular QRST isoareas are not independent of the activation sequence (Lux et al, 1980), and local ventricular recovery properties and effective refractory periods are modified instantaneously with changes in the activation sequence (Abildskov, 1976). This suggests that alterations in activation sequence associated with secondary repolarization changes also induce primary repolarization changes or that QRST isoareas do not reliably measure primary repolarization properties. Hence, we cannot accept PTa voltage-time integrals and spatial atrial gradient as absolute measures of primary repolarization properties in the atrium, but they can be considered to reflect spatial changes of repolarization (Lux et al, 1980; Herweg et al, 2001).

The protocols used to study the atrium involved pacing from the sinus node region or from the left atrial appendage using a protocol (Figure 5) similar to that in ventricle. We paced at rates 5% faster than sinus rate as well as 50% faster than sinus rate from both sites. In this way, we could isolate the effects of altering rate alone, altering activation alone, or altering both. As demonstrated in Figure 6, when right atrial pacing rate alone was increased, there was no effect on the spatial atrial gradient during either

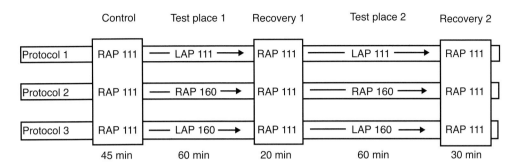

Figure 5 Experimental protocol. RAP, right atrial pacing; LAP, left atrial pacing. Numbers for RAP and LAP are beats/min. Modified with permission from Herweg et al, 2001.

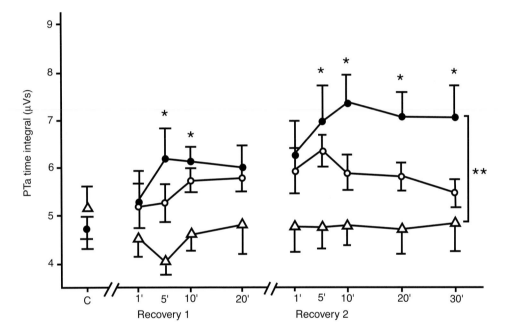

Figure 6 Spatial atrial gradient during right atrial (RA) pacing at control and in recovery periods 1 and 2 in four dogs, after two (one hour) periods of: ● pacing from the left atrial appendage (LAA) at 160 bpm (altered activation sequence and increased rate); ○ pacing from LAA with no change in rate (altered activation sequence); and △ pacing from RA at 160 bpm (increased rate without alteration in activation sequence). The spatial atrial gradient increased after pacing with an altered activation sequence at increased rate. **$P < 0.05$ by ANOVA, *$P < 0.05$ by Bonferroni's test. Modified with permission from Herweg et al, 2001.

recovery period from pacing. When activation alone was changed by pacing from the left atrium, a modest change in the spatial atrial gradient occurred. However, when rapid left atrial pacing was performed, accumulation of a change in atrial gradient occurred during both recovery periods. This was consistent with cardiac memory. Moreover, preliminary data (Chandra et al, 2000) suggest that after several days of pacing over an altered activation pathway from the left atrium there is the onset of atrial tachyarrhythmias. The etiology of these and their possible relationship to inducibility of atrial fibrillation are the subject of ongoing studies.

Discussion

Changes in the site of impulse initiation and the resultant pathway of activation frequently occur in the heart, whether as the result of arrhythmias or of pacemaker implantation. The studies referred to in this article highlight some of the events that may ensue as a result of modest changes in rate and activation pathway. The first point to be made is that simply changing the activation pathway in the heart has a profound effect on repolarization based on steps that appear to reside in mechanoelectrical coupling (Ricard et al, 1999; Sadoshima and Izumo, 1993; Sadoshima et al, 1992). This is stated because it is the alteration in the stress/strain relationship in the ventricle that appears to set off the cascade of events that induce the repolarization changes (Ricard et al, 1999). To date, signal transduction related to altered activation has been studied in ventricle only (Ricard et al, 1999; Patberg et al, 2001), and even this information is quite incomplete. Whether the angiotensin II pathway is the only one involved is not certain. Neither is it known what steps exist between the receptor and the target protein (e.g., I_{to}). Is there a change in the immediate early gene program and alteration in the synthesis of specific target proteins? Is I_{to} the only target protein? This is viewed as unlikely. That new protein synthesis is involved in the occurrence of the repolarization changes is clear (Shvilkin et al, 1998); however, the specific events that occur in protein synthesis are undefined. Information regarding the transduction pathways involved in atrium is even more rudimentary. It is obvious, however, that given the nature of the signal in atrium (the Ta wave), tracking the changes that occur is far more difficult than in ventricle (Herweg et al, 2001). Moreover, preliminary data in the atrium suggest the effect of altering activation pathway may be arrhythmogenic (Chandra et al, 2000), which does not necessarily appear to be the case in ventricle (Shvilkin et al, 1998; Plotnikov et al, 2001; Rosen, 2001). Hence, much remains to be done if the etiology of the repolarization changes in atrium and their implications for cardiac rhythm are to be understood.

Summary

The study of activation-induced changes in repolarization has a long way to go. However, as more is learned about the mechanisms determining these changes, the likelihood increases that it will be possible to deliberately manipulate activation and repolarization in ways that improve cardiac function. These manipulations have the potential for major clinical impact, as follows: first, studies to date using single, dual, or multisite pacing as therapeutic interventions in settings as diverse as hypertrophic cardiomyopathy and atrial fibrillation already suggest therapeutic potential (Delfaut et al, 1998; Foster et al, 1995; Gadler et al, 1997; Prinzen et al, 1990). Second, and more speculatively, now that the evolution of cardiac memory impacts on antiarrhythmic drug interactions with the heart is known (Plotnikov et al, 2001), it may be possible to devise protocols for drug administration that limit the propensity to proarrhythmia. Finally, exploration of induction of cardiac memory in its own right to modify repolarization and prolong refractoriness may carry the potential for direct antiarrhythmic benefit.

Acknowledgment

The studies referred to were supported in part by USPHS-NHLBI grants: HL-28958, HL-53956, HL-67101 and HL-67449.

CHAPTER 6

EFFECTS OF INCREASED HEART RATE ON CORONARY ATHEROGENESIS AND ITS REVERSAL BY BRADYCARDIA INDUCED BY SINUS NODE ABLATION OR β-ADRENERGIC BLOCKADE

THOMAS B. CLARKSON

INTRODUCTION

Although concentrations of plasma lipids and lipoproteins are major determinants of the progression of atherosclerosis, numerous studies have found that they contribute only 35%–40% to the variability seen in the extent of coronary artery atherosclerosis in both human study participants and in experimental animals. Consequently, efforts have sought to determine other major independent variables affecting atherogenesis. A number of epidemiologic studies have found a relationship between heart rate and coronary heart disease with low heart rates being associated with a lower incidence and higher heart rates with an increased incidence of the disease (Dyer et al, 1980; Kannel et al, 1987). Similarly, a number of experimental observations have indicated a heart-rate dependence for the development of coronary lesions (Beere et al, 1984; Kaplan et al, 1987a). In this chapter, the salient features of the clinical and experimental observations are discussed.

CLINICAL STUDIES

A notable contribution to understanding the relationship between heart rate and the rate of progression of angiographically demonstrable coronary atherosclerosis has been made by Perski et al (1992). In this study, the investigators followed coronary artery plaque size in men who had developed myocardial infarction at a younger age. Two subsets of 25 men in each group were selected based on their minimal heart rate (43 versus 53 beats/min). The relation of their mean heart rate and their coronary artery atherosclerosis is shown in Figure 1. The study indicated that high minimal heart rates recorded during 24-h continuous monitoring was a predictor of rapid progression of coronary atherosclerosis in young male patients after myocardial infarction.

NONHUMAN PRIMATE STUDIES

The strength of the epidemiologic association between low heart rate and low occurrence of coronary heart disease (discussed elsewhere in this monograph) has prompted studies of the phenomenon in nonhuman primate models. In an innovative experiment, Beere et al (1984) compared the quantitative extent of coronary artery atherosclerosis, and later of carotid bifurcation atherosclerosis (Beere et al, 1992), of male cynomolgus monkeys fed an atherogenic diet and that had been subjected to sinoatrial node ablation or were sham operated and had innately low heart rates. The monkeys were considered to have low heart rates at 130 beats/min and high heart rates at 150 beats/min and above. Beere et al (1984, 1992) found a large and significant difference in both coronary artery atherosclerosis and carotid bifurcation atherosclerosis between the animals with low and high heart rates (Figures 2 and 3).

The observations by Beere et al (1984) have been confirmed and extended by Kaplan et al (1987a). In their study, male cynomolgus monkeys living in social groups of five animals each and fed a moderately atherogenic diet were used. Plasma lipid and lipoprotein measurements were made, as well as

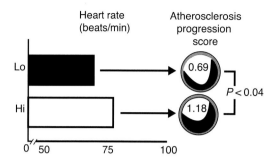

Figure 1 Effect of heart rate on coronary artery atherosclerosis progression of human males. Modified from Perski et al, 1992.

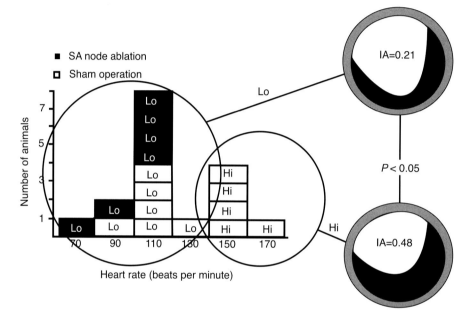

Figure 2 Effect of heart rate on coronary artery atherosclerosis (IA, intimal area or plaque area) of male cynomolgus monkeys with sinoatrial node ablation or sham operation and fed an atherogenic diet. Modified from Beere et al, 1984.

measurements of "casual" heart rates by radiotelemetry. Again, a large and statistically significant difference in coronary artery atherosclerosis plaque size was found (Figure 4). The investigators also determined whether these heart rate–related differences in the extent of coronary artery atherosclerosis might be due to differences in other more traditional risk factors such as the serum lipids and blood pressure. Of the serum lipids and blood pressure variables, only serum high-density lipoprotein cholesterol concentrations differed between the groups. The animals with high heart rates had high-density lipoprotein cholesterol concentrations of about 35 mg/dL compared with the animals in the low heart rate group with high-density lipoprotein cholesterol concentrations of about 45 mg/dL ($P < 0.02$). The atherosclerotic plaque size differences in the coronary arteries were re-examined by analysis of covariance entering the high-density lipoprotein cholesterol concentrations as a covariant. The analysis of covariance revealed that the high-density lipoprotein cholesterol concentration differences between the monkeys with high and low heart rates did not appreciably affect the association between heart rate and coronary atherosclerosis and the P value remained unchanged.

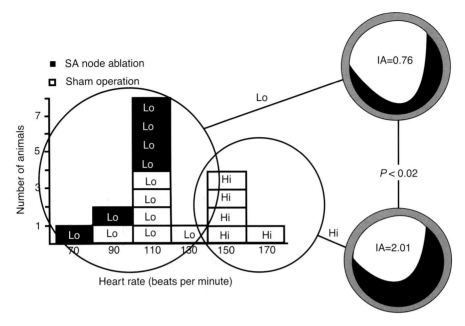

Figure 3 Effect of heart rate on carotid bifurcation atherosclerosis (IA, intimal area or plaque area) of male cynomolgus monkeys with sinoatrial node ablation or sham operation and fed an atherogenic diet. Modified from Beere et al, 1992.

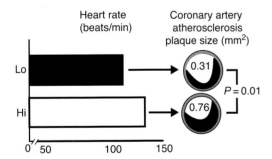

Figure 4 Effect of heart rate on the extent of coronary artery atherosclerosis of male cynomolgus monkeys fed an atherogenic diet. Modified from Kaplan et al, 1987a.

BEHAVIORAL EXACERBATION OF ATHEROSCLEROSIS IN MALE MONKEYS

Much of our understanding of the importance of increases in heart rate has evolved from studies of the behavioral exacerbation of atherosclerosis in male monkeys (Kaplan et al, 1982). In these studies, male cynomolgus monkeys were fed a moderately atherogenic diet and were housed in five-member social groups, and these social groups were assigned to two experimental conditions. One of these conditions was termed "unstable." In that condition, animals were redistributed among groups on a regular basis, and, furthermore, an estrogen-implanted female was placed into each of these groups in the latter half of each reorganization to provide an additional stimulus for inter-male competition. The remainder of the groups were in a stable condition. That condition was one in which the group memberships were maintained without disruption and without introduction of estrogenized females. Following an experimental period of about two years, the extent of coronary atherosclerosis was evaluated morphometrically. The animals housed in the unstable condition (reorganized social groups) developed about twice as much coronary atherosclerosis as animals in the stable condition but only if they were of high social rank (dominant) (Figure 5). Subordinate animals, regardless of their social situation, developed an amount of

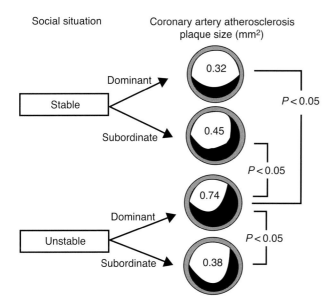

Figure 5 Coronary artery atherosclerosis extent of dominant and subordinate monkeys housed in stable and unstable (periodically reorganized) social groups. Dominant monkeys in unstable groups had more coronary artery atherosclerosis than did dominant monkeys in stable groups, and more than subordinates in either social condition ($P < 0.05$). Adapted from Kaplan et al, 1982.

coronary artery atherosclerosis generally equivalent to that of dominant animals housed in the stable condition. During the course of these studies, it became apparent that the dominant monkeys living in the unstable condition engaged in episodes such as contact aggression that markedly increased their heart rates.

In a separate study, Manuck et al (1986) sought to quantify the differences in heart rate in dominant and subordinate cynomolgus male monkeys during occurrences of different behavioral states. Using radiotelemetry, the heart rates of the male monkeys were recorded under two behavioral conditions. One of these was while monkeys were sitting alone but were within touching distance of another monkey, referred to in the studies as "close proximity." The other was when the monkeys were alone and not within touching distance of another monkey, referred to as "alone at a distance." Those observations are summarized in Figure 6. Heart rates while the monkeys were in "close proximity" were significantly lower than when the animals were sitting "alone at a distance." The difference between dominant and subordinate monkeys was small when the animals were in "close proximity." However, the heart rates were considerably greater among the dominant animals while "alone at a distance." Based on those and other observations, it was concluded that the increased heart rates of the dominant animals during various social interchanges, particularly in the unstable social situation, might be a major determinant of their exacerbated atherosclerosis.

β-ADRENERGIC BLOCKADE AND BEHAVIORAL EXACERBATION OF ATHEROSCLEROSIS IN MALE MONKEYS

To gain further insight into the role of increased heart rate in the exacerbation of coronary atherosclerosis of dominant monkeys living in a socially unstable condition, a study was conducted and reported investigating the effect of propranolol treatment on the extent of coronary artery atherosclerosis in such behaviorally predisposed monkeys fed an atherogenic diet (Kaplan et al, 1987b). In that study, male cynomolgus monkeys were maintained in social groups of five animals each. All groups were maintained under socially unstable conditions exactly as used previously. Half of the animals were "untreated" and received no β-adrenergic blocking agent. The other half of the animals were "treated" and were administered propranolol in the diet. The experiment lasted for 26 months, after which the animals underwent necropsy and the extensiveness of coronary artery atherosclerosis was evaluated morphometrically. The results of that study are presented in Figure 7. Propranolol treatment decreased the heart rates of the

Heart Rate and Atherosclerosis Progression

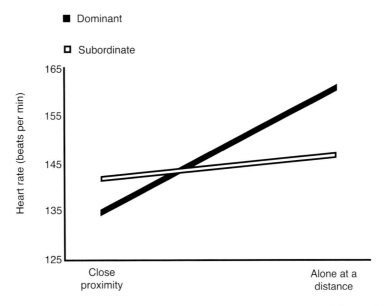

Figure 6 Mean heart rates of dominant and subordinate male monkeys recorded during different behavioral situations. Data presented are heart rates recorded when animals were in "close proximity" and "alone at a distance." Adapted from Manuck et al, 1986.

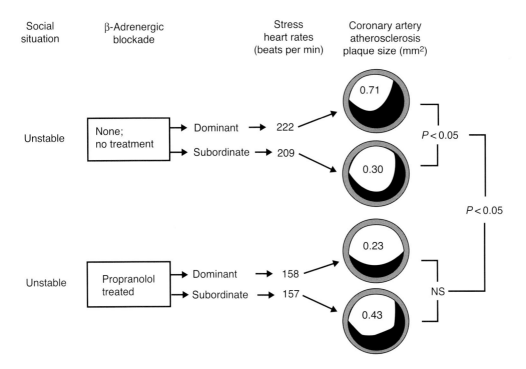

Figure 7 Coronary artery atherosclerosis extent in dominant and subordinate monkeys, all housed in unstable groups and either untreated or treated with propranolol hydrochloride. Exacerbated coronary artery atherosclerosis of dominant animals living in unstable groups was completely inhibited by β-adrenergic blockade. NS, not significant. Adapted from Kaplan et al, 1987b.

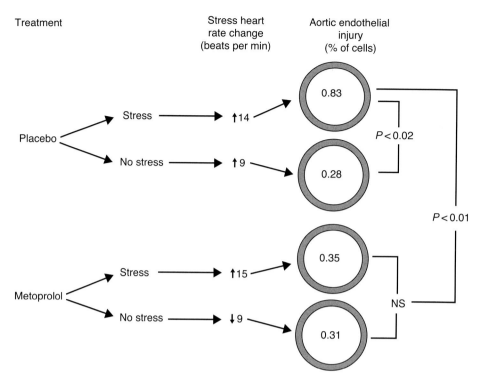

Figure 8 Proportion of injured endothelial cells in the aorta from cynomolgus monkeys stressed or not stressed and treated or not treated with a β-adrenergic blocking drug (metoprolol). Percentage of IgG-positive cells on Hautchen preparations was taken as index of arterial injury. NS, not significant. Adapted from Skantze et al, 1998.

dominant animals during stressful events in their social setting from a mean of 222 beats/min to 158 beats/min. There were also decreases in heart rates of subordinate animals from 209 to 157 beats/min with propranolol treatment. Propranolol treatment, leading to the attenuation of the elevated heart rates during the stress of the social environment, resulted in an inhibition of the behaviorally exacerbated atherosclerosis of the dominant animals with the mean plaque size measured in the coronary arteries of the dominant animals being decreased from 0.71 mm^2 to 0.26 mm^2 ($P < 0.05$). The antiatherogenic effect of propranolol on dominant animals was independent of its effects on serum plasma lipid concentrations or on blood pressure. It was concluded that prevention of increased heart rates associated with stressful environments was the mechanism by which β-adrenergic blockade inhibited the exacerbated coronary atherogenesis.

INCREASED HEART RATES AND ENDOTHELIAL DYSFUNCTION IN MONKEYS

There is now a consensus that endothelial injury and dysfunction are major events in the pathogenesis of exacerbated atherosclerosis. Endothelial dysfunction is associated with increased permeability to the plasma low-density lipoproteins, decreases in the production of nitric oxide, and an adverse modulation of adhesion molecules. Experiments have been conducted and reported that were designed to evaluate the effect of β-adrenergic blockade on the adverse effects of stress-related increases in heart rate on endothelial injury and function. The first of these studies was by Strawn et al (1991). In their protocol, untreated cynomolgus monkeys were compared with monkeys of the same species treated with a β-blocker (metoprolol), with respect to the extent of endothelial dysfunction measured following behaviorally induced increases in heart rate. Among untreated monkeys, the psychosocial stress increased heart rates from a mean of 126–164 beats/min. Stressed monkeys given metoprolol decreased their heart rates from 146–122 beats/min. The percentage of dysfunctional endothelial cells was about 1.7 cells at heart rates of 164 and only 0.6 at heart rates of 122 ($P < 0.05$).

More recently, Skantze et al (1998) conducted an additional study of endothelial injury in cynomolgus monkeys treated with a β-adrenergic blocker. In their experiments, male cynomolgus monkeys were exposed to a psychological stressor (72 h of introduction to socially strange monkeys). The monkeys were found to have a significantly higher frequency of IgG-positive (injured) endothelial cells in the descending thoracic aorta compared with control monkeys not exposed to the stressor. Pretreatment of the monkeys with a β-adrenergic blocking agent (metoprolol) prevented the development of stress-induced endothelial injury (Figure 8). It was concluded that psychosocial stress (exposure to strange monkeys) resulted in endothelial injury and that this injury could be prevented by β-adrenergic blockade. The most predominate change associated with β-adrenergic activation was the increase in heart rate.

Conclusions

The known association between low heart rate and the correspondingly lower incidence of coronary heart disease in humans has prompted studies in nonhuman primate models. For example, comparisons were made with respect to the extent of coronary artery atherosclerosis in male cynomolgus monkeys, fed an atherogenic diet, and in those in which sinoatrial node ablation or sham operation had been performed as well as in those with intrinsically low heart rates. Coronary artery atherosclerosis was consistently less among animals with low versus high heart rates. The majority of studies relating heart rate to coronary artery atherogenesis have involved "heart rate reactivity," which is the increase in heart rate following a standardized psychologic stress. Again, the extent of coronary atherosclerosis was found to be about 2- to 3-fold higher in monkeys which were high heart rate reactors compared with those which were lower heart rate reactors. Of particular importance have been the observations in a number of studies in which the effects of β-adrenergic blockade have been determined in monkeys which had the proclivity to develop enhanced atherogenesis at high heart rates. For example, in one study among untreated monkeys, the stressor increased heart rates from a mean of 126–164 beats/min. Stressed monkeys given a β-blocker decreased heart rates from 146–122 beats/min. In these, the percentage of dysfunctional endothelial cells was about 1.7 cells at heart rates of 164 beats per min and only 0.6 at heart rates of 122 beats per min ($P < 0.05$). Thus, the data presented in this brief review provide evidence that increased heart rates are associated with the increased progression of coronary artery atherosclerosis. Furthermore, they support the conclusion that the increased heart rate–induced exacerbation of coronary atherosclerosis appears to be modulated by endothelial injury and dysfunction. The adverse changes in the extent of coronary atherosclerosis and endothelial injury and dysfunction induced by accelerated heart rates were found to be reduced by heart rate reduction by sinus node ablation and by β-adrenergic blockade. Whether such a reduction may also be produced by specific heart rate lowering effects is not known but the possibility carries significant clinical implications for the treatment of coronary artery disease.

CHAPTER 7

HEART RATE AS A RISK FACTOR IN MODIFYING THE EFFECTS OF MYOCARDIAL ISCHEMIA: EXPERIMENTAL AND CLINICAL CORRELATIONS

STEPHEN F. VATNER

PHYSIOLOGICAL REGULATION OF HEART RATE

The major determinants of myocardial oxygen consumption (MVO_2) include preload, afterload (wall stress), myocardial contractility, and heart rate. Arguably, heart rate is the most important determinant. In the normal heart, an increase in MVO_2 is met primarily by an increase in coronary blood flow, since almost all O_2 is extracted across the heart, even at rest. When the heart rate is varied over a wide range, there is almost a linear relationship between heart rate and coronary blood flow (White et al, 1971) (Figure 1). Changes in preload and afterload do not generally cause such variations in coronary blood flow, unless arterial driving pressure also changes. Therefore, heart rate becomes potentially the most important determinant of MVO_2. Under normal conditions, the heart can vary its MVO_2 over a wide range and coronary blood flow can decrease or increase to meet the metabolic requirements. One of the best examples is the response of coronary blood flow to maximal exercise. In dogs running freely and spontaneously in the field, radiotelemetered measurements of coronary blood flow increased roughly fourfold, that is, in proportion to increases in heart rate (Vatner et al, 1972) (Figure 2). This is further indirect evidence of the importance of heart rate in regulating coronary blood flow and MVO_2, although increases in inotropic state and other effects of catecholamines also exert a role. Note, however, in Figure 3 that increasing heart rate by electrical stimulation to the same level as occurred during severe

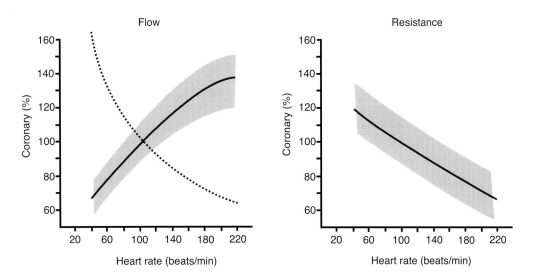

Figure 1 Left panel – Effects of stepwise changes in ventricular rate on blood flow in the left circumflex coronary artery. Broken line on coronary flow graph represents stroke coronary flow. Solid line represents average values. Shaded area indicates range of value. Right panel: mean effects on flow resistance in the coronary bed calculated from simultaneous mean arterial pressure and flow values. All results are expressed as percentage of mean value at a ventricular rate of 100 beats/min. Reproduced with permission from White et al, 1971.

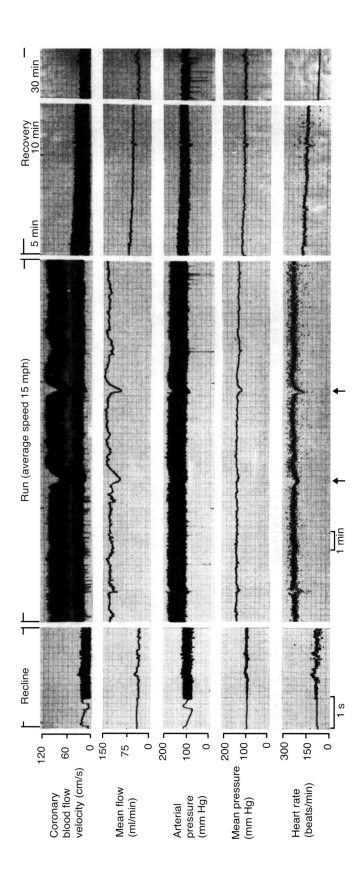

Figure 2 A typical record at rest (left panel), during extended severe exercise (middle panel), and during early and later recovery (right panel). Phasic and mean values for left circumflex coronary flow and arterial pressure and instantaneous heart rate are shown. Arrows in middle panel point to when the dog decreased running speed to change direction. Reproduced with permission from Vatner et al, 1972.

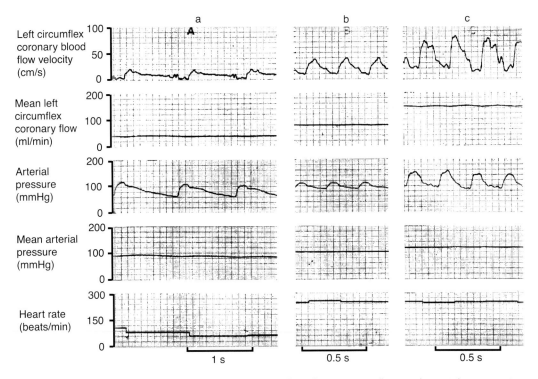

Figure 3 Comparison of phasic waveforms and mean values for coronary flow and arterial pressure in a dog at rest (a), at rest during atrial stimulation at a frequency of 248 beats/min (b), and during exercise paced at the same frequency (c). Reproduced with permission from Vatner et al, 1972.

exercise, but in the absence of increasing contractility and actually decreasing preload, is responsible for a significant fraction of the total increase in coronary blood flow during exercise.

REGULATION OF HEART RATE IN THE ISCHEMIC HEART

The situation is quite different in patients with chronic coronary artery disease, or for that matter any condition that might diminish coronary reserve, for example, hypertrophy. Coronary reserve in the normal heart allows for three to fivefold increases in coronary blood flow in response to severe exercise or maximal vasodilatation with adenosine (Vatner et al, 1972; Murray and Vatner, 1981; Hittinger et al, 1989). When coronary reserve is reduced as in coronary artery disease or myocardial hypertrophy, the metabolic stimulation of increasing heart rate either by electronic pacing or by exercise cannot be met by an appropriate increase in coronary blood flow (Murray and Vatner, 1981; Hittinger et al, 1989). This results in an imbalance between myocardial O_2 metabolic demand and supply, which induces myocardial ischemia. Therefore, in patients with reduced coronary reserve, it becomes critical to limit any increase in heart rate, and reducing it becomes advantageous as long as arterial pressure and cardiac output can be maintained.

These concepts have been translated to the clinical arena. Approximately 30 years ago, there was considerable interest in determining factors that affected the size of myocardial infarction. Despite some shortcomings in experimental design, the study by Maroko et al (1971) was a landmark. That study suggested the ECG-ST segment elevation as an index of myocardial ischemia, and clearly indicated that increased heart rate may be an adverse factor in experimental myocardial ischemia (Figure 4). With all other variables relatively constant, increasing heart rate will result in extending the ischemic damage induced by coronary artery occlusion, where reducing heart rate will have a salutary effect. This concept

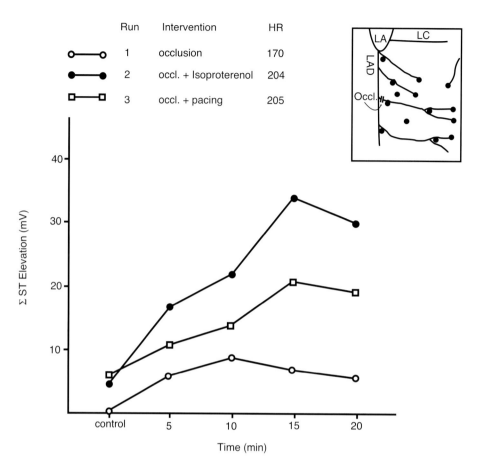

Figure 4 Effects of heart rate on ST elevation during coronary artery occlusion. Effects of tachycardia and isoproterenol. ΣST, sum of ST-segment elevations. Heart rate increased ΣST, an indirect measure of ischemic changes, and isoproterenol at the same rate, increased ΣST further. HR, heart rate; LAD, left anterior descending artery; LC, left circumflex artery. Reproduced with permission from Maroko et al, 1971.

was supported time and again in the clinical setting where it is well recognized that tachycardia or tachyarrhythmias have multiple detrimental effects in the setting of myocardial ischemia.

Indeed, chronic tachycardia can even induce heart failure in the normal heart (Shinbane et al, 1997), and a brief tachycardic stimulation can hasten and intensify the development of heart failure in an already diseased heart. Thus, it is not difficult to understand how deleterious tachycardia can be in patients with limited coronary reserve and with acute or chronic myocardial ischemia. Conversely, reducing the heart rate has repeatedly been shown to be advantageous. Perhaps the best example is with cold cardioplegia where not only lowering the temperature of the heart, but also its rate, renders the heart substantially more resistant to ischemic heart damage (Van Camp et al, 1995).

At about the time that it was becoming appreciated that increasing MVO_2 may be a problem for patients with acute ischemia, there was still an effort by pharmaceutical companies to develop synthetic sympathomimetic amines as potential therapy for heart failure, and even myocardial ischemia. The goal of these efforts was to develop agents that increased contractility in the absence of a change in heart rate or pressure. Most of these agents have been discontinued for chronic use, since clinical trials have generally found that outcomes are worsened with extended periods of administration, even if there is an initial positive effect. It is interesting to speculate that a different approach, an increase in contractility in the absence of changes in heart rate or pressure, and independent of β-adrenergic stimulation, may have been

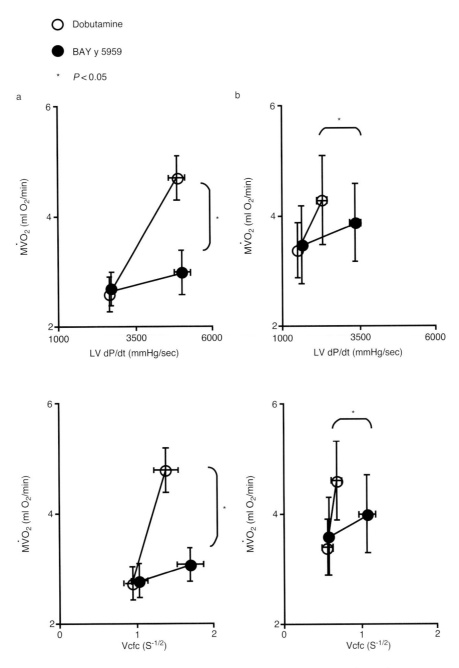

Figure 5 Effects of dobutamine (10 μg/kg/min) and BAY y 5959, a calcium channel promoter, (210 μg/kg/min) on the relation between myocardial oxygen consumption (MVO_2) and either dP/dt (top; $n = 9$) or V_{cfc} (bottom; $n = 8$) in conscious dogs before (a) and after (b) pacing-induced heart failure. Before heart failure, BAY y 5959 and dobutamine resulted in similar increases in left ventricular (LV) dP/dt and V_{cfc}, but the increase in MVO_2 with BAY y 5959 was significantly smaller than with dobutamine ($P < 0.05$). After heart failure, the relationship between MVO_2 and either LV dP/dt or V_{cfc} remained unchanged for both dobutamine and BAY y 5959. Increases in LV dP/dt and V_{cfc} with BAY y 5959 were significantly greater than with dobutamine ($P < 0.05$), whereas the increase in MVO_2 with BAY y 5959 was slightly but significantly smaller than with dobutamine. All data are mean ± SE. Reproduced with permission from Asai et al, 1998.

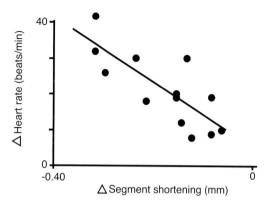

Figure 6 The relationship between increases in heart rate (ordinate) and decreases in segment shortening rate (ordinate) in severely ischemic segments is shown. The linear regression was significant, $P < 0.01$, $r = 0.79$. Reproduced with permission from Vatner et al, 1979.

more positive. Indeed, preliminary evidence suggests that increasing Ca^{2+} availability may have a positive effect in experimental heart failure (Asai et al, 1998) (Figure 5).

The importance of heart rate in determining the consequences of administering sympathomimetic amines in acute myocardial ischemia was also studied in our laboratory (Vatner and Baig, 1979). In these experiments, three different sympathomimetic amines (isoproterenol, dopamine, and dobutamine) were compared under conditions of either increasing heart rate or heart rate held constant. Isoproterenol exerts potentially the most severe deleterious effects in the ischemic setting because it not only increases contractility, but also increases heart rate in the face of declining arterial pressure. It turns out that the decrease in pressure is critical, because it elicits a "coronary steal," which shifts blood flow from ischemic to normal tissue. In that study, experiments were conducted with matched inotropic conditions, both when heart rate was allowed to increase or was held constant (Vatner and Baig, 1979). Several interesting points were uncovered. First, when all the data were plotted, a good correlation was observed between decreases in myocardial segmental shortening, that is, an adverse effect on regional myocardial contraction, versus increases in heart rate (Figure 6), indicating a potent negative effect of increasing heart rate on regional ischemic myocardial contraction. The other interesting conclusions are derived from the accompanying table (Table 1). Again with matched increases in contractility, all sympathomimetic amines exerted a deleterious effect on ischemic zone blood flow and function as long as heart rate rose. When heart rate was held constant, the negative effects were less apparent, and there was actually a potentially positive outcome with dopamine. Thus, all sympathomimetic amines that increase myocardial contractility do not necessarily exert negative effects in the ischemic setting, and in particular, do not exert a "coronary steal" as long as heart rate does not rise. However, when inotropic stimulation is coupled with either tachycardia or hypotension in the ischemic heart, the effects of ischemia are intensified, in part, through "coronary steal" mechanisms.

It is important to keep in mind that the take-home message from these types of studies is not so straightforward as was thought 20–30 years ago. Now it is recognized that many of these types of interventions that affect heart rate and myocardial contractility, even relatively acutely, not only will exert an action directly on the myocardium, but can also affect the genomic expression in the heart as well as induce changes in proteins. Importantly, β-adrenergic stimulation affects a host of primary, secondary, and tertiary signaling pathways, not only including protein kinase A (PKA) and cyclic adenosine monophosphate (cAMP) but also stress-activated proteins. These other pathways may actually be responsible for some of the deleterious effects of sympathomimetic amine stimulation, independent of changes in MVO_2 or coronary blood flow (Homcy et al, 1991).

There are other indirect effects of heart rate, which have been reported to exert a negative effect on chronic ischemic heart disease. Indeed, it has been suggested that heart rate affects both the vascular structure and myocardium. Tachycardia impairs vascular compliance and can even accelerate atherogenesis (Perski et al, 1992). For vascular function, arterial mechanical properties are determined by elastic, viscous, and inertial components of the vessel wall. Arterial stiffness is frequency dependent (Mangoni et al, 1996). In experimental studies, pacing-induced tachycardia is associated with reductions in arterial

TABLE 1. Effects of heart rate on responses of sympathomimetic amines in myocardial ischemia

	ISO (0.03)	DP (4)	DP (10)* (T)	DP (10)* (NT)	DB (4)	DB (10)* (T)	DB (10)* (NT)
LV dP/dt	+	+	+++	+++	+	+++	+++
Mean arterial pressure	–	0	+	+	0	+	+
Heart Rate	++	0	++	0	0	++	0
Normal zone resistance	– –	–	–	– –	– –	–	–
Ischemic zone blood flow	–	0	–	+	0	–	0

+, increase; –, decrease; 0, no significant change; ISO, isoproterenol; DP, dopamine; DB, dobutamine; T, tachycardia; NT, no tachycardia. * The same dose of dopamine or dobutamine caused a decrease in ischemic zone blood flow, when heart rate rose (T), as was also observed with isoproterenol, which increased heart rate.

compliance and distensibility (Mangoni et al, 1996). Sa Cunha et al (1997) also showed a positive correlation between high heart rate and increased arterial stiffness in hypertensive patients.

Heart rate can also alter the progression of atherogenesis. Beere et al demonstrated that reduction in heart rate by sinus node ablation delayed the onset of coronary and carotid atheroma in monkeys fed an atherogenic diet when compared with a sham group (Beere et al, 1984, 1992). The relationship between heart rate and accelerated atherogenesis is explained either by differences in vascular mechanics or by lipid profiles. The pulsatile nature of the blood flow causes local hemodynamic effects and the oscillations in the direction of wall shear stress prolong the stagnation of blood particles, thereby increasing the time for blood vessel-wall interaction. Hemodynamic stress fluctuations are mainly observed during systole. In addition, a positive correlation was reported between the resting heart rate and lipid abnormalities (Bonaa and Arnesen, 1992), although there is a possibility that it is induced by catecholamines influencing cardiac hemodynamics and lipid metabolism.

Indeed, epidemiologic studies have shown that a high heart rate at rest is a risk factor for cardiovascular mortality, which can be independent from the acute consequences of tachycardia on myocardial metabolism (Dyer et al, 1980; Kannel et al, 1987; Shaper et al, 1993), but most importantly, it aggravates the symptoms of myocardial ischemia by increasing metabolic demand, particularly in the face of limited coronary reserve.

Finally, increased heart rate is an ominous prognostic sign in the setting of myocardial infarction. On the one hand, tachycardia sometimes contributes to the development of lethal ventricular tachyarrhythmias and sudden cardiac death by decreasing the ventricular fibrillation threshold (Myers et al, 1974; James et al, 1977; Parker et al, 1990; Aupetit et al, 1998). In addition, heart rate variability and heart rate turbulence relate to the prognosis of the patients with coronary arterial disease. Thus, heart rate, by itself, seems to be a true cardiovascular risk factor and agents that improve the coronary circulation or enhance cardiac output in the absence of increasing heart rate are more advantageous to patients with heart disease than those that also elicit tachycardia.

SUMMARY

The major determinants of myocardial oxygen consumption (MVO_2) include preload, afterload (wall stress), myocardial contractility, and heart rate, with heart rate potentially the most important determinant. In the normal heart, an increase in MVO_2 is met primarily by an increase in coronary blood flow. When heart rate is varied over a wide range, there is almost a linear relationship between heart rate and coronary blood flow. The situation is quite different in patients with chronic coronary artery disease, or for that matter, any condition that might diminish coronary reserve, for example, hypertrophy. When coronary reserve is reduced as in coronary artery disease, the metabolic stimulation of increasing heart rate either by electronic pacing or by exercise cannot be met by an appropriate increase in coronary blood flow. This results in an imbalance between myocardial O_2 metabolic demand and supply, which induces or exacerbates myocardial ischemia. Increasing heart rate by electrical stimulation can be used as a test for latent coronary artery disease, that is, pacing-induced angina. Tachycardia will also extend myocardial ischemic damage during myocardial infarction within any given area at risk. Conversely, lowering heart rate exerts a protective effect in the ischemic setting. Therefore, in patients with reduced coronary reserve, it becomes critical to limit any increase in heart rate, and reducing it becomes advantageous as long as arterial pressure and cardiac output can be maintained.

Acknowledgment

This study was supported in part by HL33107, HL33065, HL59139, HL62442, HL65182, HL65183, HL69020 and AG14121.

CHAPTER 8

BRADYCARDIA AND HEART RATE VARIABILITY

Jean Yves Le Heuzey and Xavier Copie

Introduction

Heart rate and heart rate variability are major prognostic factors in many cardiovascular disorders. Although these two parameters are closely linked, they each provide somewhat differing information. Sinus bradycardia is due to changes in the electrophysiologic properties of sinus node cells. These changes correspond to intrasinus pacemaker shifts with modifications in the site of emergence of the excitation wave. Many vagosympathetic stimuli can induce intrasinus pacemaker shifts and change the sinus rate. Positive chronotropic stimuli shift the dominant pacemaker towards the head of the sinus node, while negative chronotropic stimuli shift it towards the tail. The variations in sinus rate induced by changes in vagosympathetic tone may be assessed by the measurement of heart rate variability on Holter recordings. Time domain, frequency domain, and nonlinear analysis methods have been proposed to evaluate heart rate variability. Heart rate and heart rate variability are linked by a mathematical relationship but some methods are able to evaluate heart rate variability at given heart rates. Heart rate variability is of major prognostic value in many cardiac disorders such as coronary artery disease, especially postinfarction, and congestive heart failure. Drugs inducing heart rate reduction such as β-blockers are able to increase heart rate variability, especially in patients with heart failure. To date it has not been clearly demonstrated that improving heart rate variability per se may directly lead to an improvement in patient prognosis. Therefore, as yet the use of modifications of heart rate variability as a surrogate end point in clinical trials may be premature and must await the outcome of controlled clinical trials.

There is now much data which suggest that heart rate (Kannel et al, 1987, Hjalmarson et al, 1990) as well as heart rate variability (Malik, 1995) are significant prognostic factors for predicting mortality and morbidity in a number of cardiovascular disorders. However, while the two parameters are closely linked, they do not provide identical predictive information in every subset of patients with cardiac disease. Indeed, heart rate variability increases when heart rate decreases but different techniques, including Poincaré diagrams (Copie et al, 1996b) for example, are able to analyze heart rate variability for different heart rates. Heart rate variability is related largely to the autonomic nervous system tone, and heart rate, in itself, is related both to the autonomic tone as well as to intrinsic sinus node function. An understanding of the basis for the origin of the heart beat in the mammalian sinus node is the key to comprehension of heart rate modulation as a therapeutic maneuver. A discussion of the current mechanisms of the origin of the heart beat is therefore the preamble to the rest of this chapter.

Physiology of the sinus node: mechanism of bradycardia

Bradycardia may have several pathological causes: atrioventricular block, sinoatrial block including junctional escape, and frequent extrasystoles with pauses, but the main cause of bradycardia is the slowing of sinus rate. This sinus bradycardia may be due to intrinsic sinus node dysfunction or to the extrinsic effects of the vagosympathetic system or both.

Anatomic-electrophysiological considerations

Located under the epicardium of the right atrium, at the junction between the superior vena cava and the right atrial appendage, the sinus node is 15–20 mm long. It is composed of cellular clusters separated by collagen and elastin fibers. The most specific cells are called P cells. They are mainly located in the head of the sinus node. Transitional fusiform cells called T cells are located at the junction with atrial fibers. Cellular junctions are few in number or lacking in the central cephalic area of the sinus node, being more abundant towards the periphery. The sympathetic and parasympathetic innervation is rich. Thus,

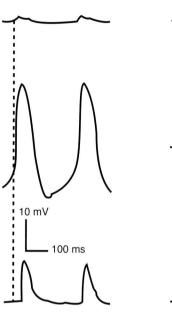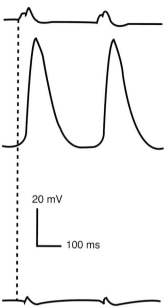

Figure 1 Recording by microelectrode of an action potential from the sinus node in isolated sinoatrial rabbit preparation. On the left, cephalic recording: dominant pacemaker; on the right, recording in the tail: latent pacemaker. The recordings in the top panel correspond to the sinus electrogram. The recordings in the bottom panel correspond to the electrograms of the crista terminalis.

the sinus node is very sensitive to nervous, hemodynamic, and humoral stimuli: sympathetic, parasympathetic, pressure, temperature, pH, O_2, CO_2, ion concentrations, cooling, and circulating hormones.

Various electrophysiological characteristics closely correspond with this very heterogeneous anatomical structure (Bleeker et al, 1980). For example, the morphologies of the cellular action potentials change relative to the sites of microelectrode recordings (Figure 1). Phase 4 of the spontaneous diastolic depolarization is very striking in the central cephalic cells. In these cells, the total amplitude of the action potential is weak as is the diastolic depolarization (–60 mV). Consequently, automaticity here is very high but intercellular conduction is very poor. In contrast, in the periphery of the sinus node, phase 4 is less marked, phase 0 is more abrupt, and the amplitude of the action potential increases; the peripheral cells of the tail of the node have a less marked degree of automaticity but the conduction of the excitation wave is more rapid than that in the cephalic central cells.

Synchronization of cellular activation and pacemaker shifts

The pacemaker cells are able to synchronize in order to produce sinus electrical activity that is regular without an extrinsic stimulus. These phenomena of cellular synchronization have been studied by many investigators (Clay and De Haan, 1979; Malik, 1995). The synchronization of the pacemaker cells is mainly due to an electrotonic conduction mechanism.

Organic alterations of several cell groups of the sinus node may be responsible for a shift of the site of origin of the cardiac excitation inside the sinus node itself or to a peripheral site. But in fact such an intrasinus pacemaker shift may be also observed in the normal sinus node under the influence of many factors such as sympathetic or parasympathetic stimulation, acetylcholine and norepinephrine, cooling, increases in potassium concentration, and decreases in calcium concentration (Le Heuzey et al, 1982, 1986). An example of this intrasinus pacemaker shift under the effect of cooling is shown in Figure 2.

These shifts in the site of origin of the cells taking over the effective control of the electrical activation in the sinus node correlate with the observed changes in sinus rate. Factors that lead to a shift of the dominant pacemaker towards the cephalic area (sympathetic stimulation, norepinephrine) bring about an increase in the sinus rate. In contrast, factors inducing a shift towards the tail of the sinus node are responsible for decreases in the sinus rate. This is the case with vagal stimulation, acetylcholine, cooling, increases in potassium concentration, and decreases in calcium concentration.

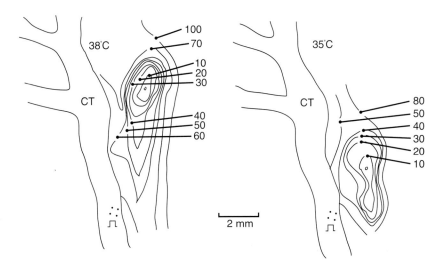

Figure 2 Shift, under the effect of temperature, of the site of excitation origin (dominant pacemaker) in rabbit sinus node. On the left, preparation at 38°C, on the right at 35°C: intrasinus pacemaker shift towards the tail of the sinus node.

These intrasinus pacemaker shifts have been confirmed in isolated sinus node preparations but also in the in situ dog heart and in humans by direct endocavity recordings of sinoatrial activity and indirectly during assessment of sinoatrial conduction.

These physiological shifts of the dominant sinus pacemaker, with a point of emergence of the excitation wave from the head or the tail of the sinus node according to a rapid or slow sinus rate, may be observed on a surface electrocardiogram, especially in young subjects with a normal sinus node stimulated by marked changes in the intensity of the vagosympathetic tone. Indeed, the axis of the P wave may change as the duration of the wave is modified: this axis is vertical and the duration is short when the emergence is in the head of the sinus node and the sinus rate is rapid. On the other hand, when the sinus cycle is long, the emergence of the excitation is in the tail of the sinus node (Figure 3). By analyzing the variations in the sinus cycles, it is possible to evaluate the changes induced by the vagosympathetic tone.

MEASUREMENT OF HEART RATE VARIABILITY

Heart rate variability permits the evaluation of the effects of autonomic nervous system influences on the cardiovascular system. Indeed, the autonomic nervous system plays a major role in the genesis of cardiac arrhythmias. Furthermore, the predictive value of heart rate variability in the postinfarction period has been demonstrated for 10 years (Kleiger et al, 1987).

Methods

It is now increasingly clear that heart rate variability may be one of the major prognostic indices in patients after myocardial infarction and in those with congestive heart failure, and possibly also in the general population (Tsuji et al, 1994). Heart rate variability may also be of value in the exploration of diabetic neuropathies (Malik, 1995). Finally, it may be of therapeutic interest to study the changes in heart rate variability induced by the effects of drugs, especially cardiovascular drugs.

Heart rate variability is usually assessed on 24-h Holter recordings. The software that is used in such studies eliminates artifacts and extrasystoles associated with the preceding and succeeding cycles.

Three types of methods may be used to assess heart rate variability: time domain, frequency domain, and nonlinear analyses.

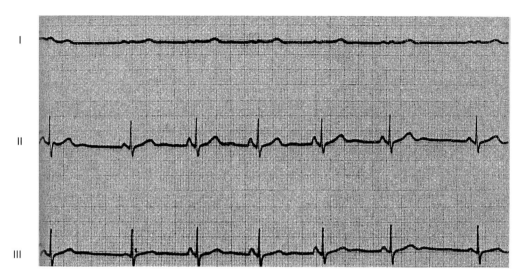

Figure 3 Variation in axis and morphology of the P wave according to the instantaneous sinus rate in a normal heart.

Time domain
The time domain analysis of heart rate variability may be undertaken by a statistical or geometric approach. The statistical approach uses the calculation of indices reflecting the dispersion of RR intervals over the duration of the recordings. It is possible to calculate the SDNN (standard deviation of all normal RR intervals) and the SDANN (standard deviation of normal RR intervals calculated for five minutes). The SDNN is one of the best parameters to stratify the risk of mortality in different populations. Other parameters are able to measure the beat-to-beat variability: RMSSD (root mean square of successive differences) and pNN50 (percentage of adjacent RR differences higher than 50 ms). These indices reflect the effect of the parasympathetic system and the vagal tone.

The geometric approach for heart rate variability has been developed by the group at St George's Hospital in London (Malik, 1995). The triangular index, also called the St George's index, is based on the analysis of RR histograms (Figure 4). Like the SDNN, the St George's index is a measure of global variability which does not allow an accurate analysis of the physiology of the autonomic nervous system. Nevertheless, it is one of the best indices to stratify the risk of mortality after myocardial infarction.

Frequency domain
The value of the analysis in the frequency domain stems from its capacity to allow an evaluation of the variability for given heart rates (Figure 5). The frequency power may be divided into different components: high frequency (0.15–0.40 Hz) and low frequency (0.04–0.15 Hz). The high-frequency component is a good estimation of the vagal tone. It is necessary to limit the use of such a method to short recordings made under standardized conditions.

Nonlinear analysis
Nonlinear analysis methods permit the description of systems with a chaotic behaviour. A simple way to attempt the assessment of these phenomena has been proposed by Henri Poincaré. The Poincaré diagram is drawn by plotting each RR interval with the preceding one (Copie et al, 1996b). Woo et al demonstrated that the shape of the Poincaré diagram was different in healthy volunteers compared with those in patients with congestive heart failure (Woo et al, 1992). To allow an accurate evaluation of this diagram, we have developed a method to assess the measurement of its width at different levels of heart rate. The dispersion in the width of the Poincaré diagram is correlated with the indices of beat-to-beat

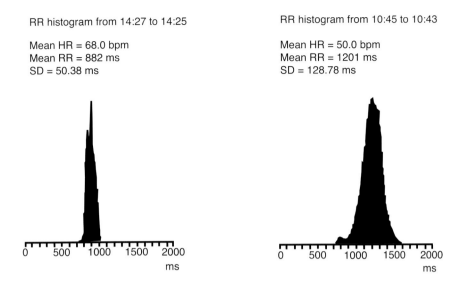

Figure 4 Histograms of normal RR intervals for 24-h Holter recordings. On these histograms, the abscissa is the duration of RR intervals and the ordinate is the number of RR intervals for each duration. When this histogram is narrow, the heart rate variability is low. On the left, low heart rate variability (SDNN = 50 ms); on the right, higher heart rate variability (SDNN = 129 ms). HR, heart rate; SD, standard deviation; SDNN, standard deviation of normal RR intervals.

variability reflecting the intensity of the vagal tone. This method allows the sampling of the vagal tone at different levels of heart rate, which is not possible with the other methods (Figure 6).

Clinical implications

Heart rate variability and coronary artery disease

Following a myocardial infarction, it has been clearly established that heart rate variability is a major prognostic factor. It has been shown in the analysis of findings in two large databases: MPIP (Multicenter Post Infarction Program) and the database of St George's Hospital in London. More recently, analysis of 24-h recordings in the Gruppo Italiano per lo Studio della Sopravvivenza nell'Infarto miocardico II (GISSI II) trial has confirmed the importance of heart rate variability in determining the risk of mortality in patients with myocardial infarction and following thrombolytic treatment (Zuanetti et al, 1996).

The significance of the prognostic value of heart rate variability has been demonstrated in the publication of Kleiger in 1987 (Kleiger et al, 1987). In this work, the authors showed that the standard deviation of normal RR intervals (SDNN) was a major prognostic factor after myocardial infarction. They analyzed the Holter recordings of 808 patients of the MPIP trial and demonstrated that an SDNN lower than 50 ms was associated with a mortality of 40% at four years, whereas the mortality of the patients with an SDNN higher than 100 ms was only 10%. Furthermore, Kleiger et al demonstrated that the heart rate variability was a factor independent of the other clinical parameters of left ventricular dysfunction, left ventricular ejection fraction, and other parameters of the Holter recordings, such as premature ventricular beats and salvoes.

Finally, it has also been demonstrated that patients with coronary artery disease but without myocardial infarction may also have impaired heart rate variability (Rich et al, 1988).

Heart rate variability and congestive heart failure

The second domain in which the study of heart rate variability may be useful is congestive heart failure. It has been shown that the main parameters of heart rate variability are also decreased in patients with

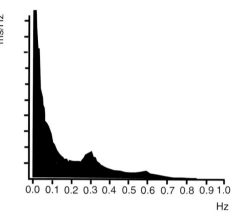

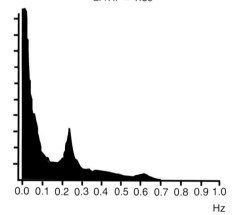

Figure 5 Spectral analysis in a patient with myocardial infarction, with normal heart rate variability. The lower spectrum was recorded in the nocturnal period and clearly shows a high frequency peak related to respiration and mediated by the parasympathetic system. FFT, fast Fourier transform; HF, high frequency; LF, low frequency; P, power; T, total.

congestive heart failure. This has been demonstrated not only for the time domain (Casolo et al, 1989) but also for the frequency domain (Saul et al, 1988). These data have been confirmed on a large scale in the UK Heart study (Nolan et al, 1998). Woo et al have demonstrated that the morphological classification of Poincaré diagrams permits the identification of the patients with congestive heart failure and a risk of sudden death (Woo et al, 1992). They described different shapes of the Poincaré diagrams: comet-shaped (normal subject), torpedo-shaped (decrease in vagal tone at all levels of heart rate), or complex shape (subjects with a high risk). These changes in the shapes of the Poincaré diagram are correlated with

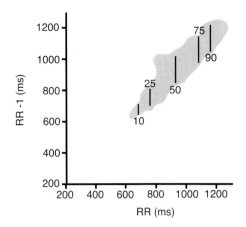

Figure 6 Measures of Poincaré diagram for different levels of heart rate. The width of the diagram is correlated to pNN50. It is a measure of beat-to-beat variability for different levels of heart rate.

the plasma catecholamine levels (Woo et al, 1994). Another group has confirmed the prognostic value of this morphological classification for the prognosis of heart failure (Brouwer et al, 1996).

The effects of drugs on heart rate variability in congestive heart failure have also been extensively studied. Thus, angiotensin-converting enzyme (ACE) inhibitors (Binkley et al, 1993) and digitalis (Krum et al, 1995) increase heart rate variability in congestive heart failure patients.

Relationship between heart rate variability and heart rate reduction

There is a direct and mathematical relationship between heart rate and heart rate variability (Copie et al, 1996a). Indeed, heart rate variability increases when heart rate decreases and vice versa. Nevertheless, as previously described, methods such as the Poincaré diagram are able to assess heart rate variability for given levels of heart rate.

The relationship between heart rate variability and bradycardia was studied in the Cardiac Insufficiency BIsoprolol Study (CIBIS I) (CIBIS Investigators and Committees, 1994). Fifty-four patients from this randomized, double-blind, placebo-controlled study were included in a heart rate variability study. The goal of this trial was to demonstrate the efficacy of a β-blocker, bisoprolol, in patients with congestive heart failure. The bisoprolol dose was 5 mg once daily. Heart rate variability was assessed during 24-h Holter recordings before randomization and after two months of treatment. Heart rate variability was measured in the time domain by the root mean square successive differences (RMSSD), the percentage of adjacent RR differences higher than 50 ms (pNN 50), and the standard deviation of RR intervals (SDNN), and in the frequency domain by high frequency (0.16–0.40 Hz) and low frequency (0.04–0.15 Hz) powers. Most patients were in New York Heart Association functional class III. The mean left ventricular ejection fraction was $27 \pm 7\%$ and heart failure was idiopathic or ischemic in half the patients. After two months, the patients receiving bisoprolol had a reduced mean heart rate compared with that of placebo patients ($P = 0.0004$). Bisoprolol increased the 24-h RMSSD ($P = 0.04$) and 24-h pNN50 ($P = 0.04$), daytime SDNN ($P = 0.05$), and daytime high frequency power ($P = 0.03$). Bisoprolol induced a significant increase in heart rate variability parameters related to parasympathetic activity in heart failure (Pousset et al, 1996). Increased vagal tone may contribute to the protective effect of β-blockers and may have prognostic implications.

In these series, Poincaré diagrams were also studied. These geometric measurements of scatterplots were used to determine beat-to-beat dispersion for different RR intervals. After two months of treatment, bisoprolol significantly increased beat-to-beat variability at the longest RR intervals ($P < 0.05$); however, there was no change in scatterplot dispersion at the shortest RR intervals (Copie et al, 1996c). This suggests that β-blockade increases parasympathetic tone or decreases sympathetic tone or both in heart failure patients only at the slowest heart rates (Figure 7).

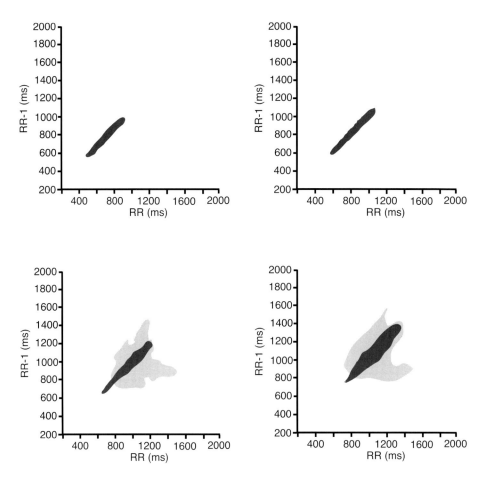

Figure 7 Holter substudy of the CIBIS I trial. Scatterplot evolution in a patient who received placebo (top) and a patient who received bisoprolol (bottom). On the left, baseline diagram; on the right, diagram after two months of treatment. Note the increase in heart rate variability with bisoprolol.

Thus, β-blocker therapy has the propensity to induce a slowing in heart rate and concomitantly to increase heart rate variability. This may be due to a mathematical relationship between heart rate and heart rate variability. In fact, it was demonstrated that part of this increase in heart rate variability may also be independent of heart rate itself.

Currently, there are no data, to our knowledge, about the effects of specific heart rate lowering agents on heart rate variability. By decreasing heart rate, these agents may induce an increase in heart rate variability but this must await the outcome of formal controlled studies. Indeed, it should be emphasized that heart rate and heart rate variability are not independent factors. To date, it has not been clearly demonstrated that improving heart rate variability itself necessarily leads to an improvement in the prognosis in patients with myocardial infarction or congestive heart failure. For these reasons, it is not yet possible to use modifications of heart rate variability as a surrogate end point in clinical trials.

CHAPTER 9

Pathophysiology of Chronic and Acute Myocardial Ischemia

Prediman K. Shah

Introduction

Myocardial ischemia is one of the major consequences of occlusive atherosclerotic coronary artery disease resulting in clinical syndromes such as stable angina, unstable angina, and silent or painless ischemia. Myocardial ischemia results from a decrease in myocardial blood flow relative to the myocardial metabolic requirements. Many episodes of ischemia are not accompanied by symptoms (silent ischemia) and, in symptomatic cases, the severity and frequency of clinical manifestations vary considerably. Even in the same patient, some episodes of ischemia may remain clinically silent, whereas others are accompanied by symptoms. In some patients, myocardial ischemia may presage a more serious clinical event such as acute myocardial infarction or sudden cardiac death. In ischemic heart disease, reduction in the frequency and severity of ischemia along with reduction in the risk of myocardial infarction and death remain the primary goals of therapeutic interventions. Over past decades, understanding of the pathophysiology of myocardial ischemia has improved with the recognition that ischemia is often the outcome of a dynamic interaction between the atherosclerotic plaque, vasomotor tone, and superimposed platelet-fibrin thrombus formation that together contribute to episodic compromise in coronary blood flow in the setting of stable and unstable ischemic heart disease. In this chapter, some of the important pathophysiologic principles of myocardial ischemia will be briefly reviewed.

Atherosclerotic plaque and luminal narrowing

A flow-limiting stenosis narrowing the coronary luminal cross-sectional area by >50%–75% in one or more epicardial coronary arteries is present in the vast majority of patients with symptomatic or painless ischemia (Campbell et al, 1985). Luminal stenosis results from the growth of atherosclerotic plaque and constrictive remodeling of adventitia. In rare cases, ischemia may occur from primary vasomotor dysfunction involving epicardial arteries with minimal or no angiographically demonstrable baseline luminal stenosis or from vasomotor dysfunction occurring at the level of the microcirculation. Epicardial coronary artery constriction or spasm is responsible for the syndrome of Prinzmetal's variant angina whereas microvascular dysfunction is thought to play a role in ischemia in patients with hypertrophic heart disease with a reduced flow reserve.

The angiographic appearance of coronary stenosis varies in terms of smoothness or irregularity of edges, length of the stenosis, presence of overhanging margins and filling defects, and concentric versus eccentric location. In general, the stenoses responsible for acute ischemic syndromes as opposed to stable coronary artery disease tend to be more complex with irregular or overhanging margins, intraluminal haziness, and filling defects occurring in 70%–80% of cases (Ambrose et al, 1985). These angiographic features are consistent with a fissured/ruptured plaque with or without a superimposed thrombus as demonstrated by angioscopic and anatomic findings (Sherman et al, 1986).

Supply–demand imbalance in ischemia

Cardiac oxygen requirements are determined by heart rate, contractility, and chamber wall stress (directly related to volume and pressure and inversely related to wall thickness). The oxygen consumption of a beating canine heart is about 8–15 mL/min/100 g of tissue. Myocardial oxygen consumption is also influenced by the fraction of energy derived from the metabolism of fatty acids, which in turn varies directly with circulating levels of fatty acids and inversely with glucose concentration. Delivery of oxygen to the heart is primarily related to coronary blood flow which is determined by the driving pressure within the coronary arteries and inversely to the coronary vascular resistance and cardiac compressive forces. Coronary vascular resistance, in turn, is regulated by metabolic, neurohormonal, and endothelial factors. Since myocardium is dominantly an aerobic organ with high oxygen extraction at rest, increases in myocardial oxygen requirements in a normal heart are matched by increases in coronary blood flow. Increased coronary blood flow in response to increased oxygen requirements results from vasodilation attributed to increased production of adenosine and other vasoactive substances such as nitric oxide (Rossen et al, 1994; Yamabe et al, 1992). Subendocardium of the left ventricle receives its blood flow predominantly during diastole, because contraction during each systole has a throttling effect that precludes substantial flow through the subendocardium. In the presence of left ventricular outflow tract obstruction where the ventricular compressive force is increased, tachycardia with shortening of diastole and relative lengthening of systole or arteriolar vasodilation induced by exercise or drugs may precipitate subendocardial ischemia even in the absence of luminal stenosis. On the other hand, normal right ventricular perfusion is systolic and diastolic because of a lower systolic pressure in the right heart. However, with right ventricular systolic hypertension, the right ventricle becomes more susceptible to ischemic damage.

Coronary blood flow has been shown to remain constant over a wide range of coronary driving pressures and distal to mild and moderate coronary stenoses under resting conditions (autoregulation) because of microvascular vasodilation. Thus, microvascular vasodilation tends to maintain normal blood flow in the presence of epicardial coronary stenosis until the stenosis becomes severe enough to exhaust autoregulatory flow reserve; at that point, any further increase in stenosis or drop in driving pressure results in a decrease in downstream blood flow (Gould et al, 1974; Gould, 1985; Freudenberg and Lichtlen, 1981; Schwartz and Bache, 1985). Since coronary collaterals do not exhibit autoregulation, flow through collaterals varies directly with the driving pressure (Kanazawa, 1994; Schaper, 1993). Coronary flow autoregulation has been attributed to both endothelium-derived nitric oxide and to direct myogenic control (Lerman and Burnett, 1992; Harrison, 1996).

METABOLIC AND FUNCTIONAL CHANGES DURING ISCHEMIA

Ischemia leads to a number of biochemical events in the myocardium that include a rapid depletion of myocardial high-energy phosphates and ADP breakdown leading to the formation of adenosine, inosine, hypoxanthine, and xanthine, a decrease in myocardial pH, and accumulation of extracellular potassium level, reduced free fatty acid extraction, reduced lactate extraction, and increased lactate production. Eventually, with severe ischemia, cellular homeostasis is lost, leading to increased intracellular calcium accumulation and irreversible myocyte damage. Ischemia results in a rapid loss of contractile function along with impairment of diastolic relaxation and increased diastolic stiffness within the ischemic segment (Steenbergen et al, 1985; Yamanishi et al, 1988). These are followed by electrocardiographic changes and, eventually, symptoms of angina; however, angina may not follow all episodes of myocardial ischemia. During regional myocardial ischemia, nonischemic segments may demonstrate compensatory hyperfunction that can attenuate decline in global ventricular function (Yamanishi et al, 1988).

PATHOGENESIS OF MYOCARDIAL ISCHEMIA: ROLE OF FIXED AND DYNAMIC STENOSIS

Myocardial ischemia in coronary artery disease results from an imbalance between myocardial energy requirements (myocardial oxygen demand) and myocardial oxygen and substrate delivery (myocardial oxygen supply) (Figure 1). In the stable phase of obstructive coronary artery disease, in which ischemia occurs mostly during physical or emotional stress, increases in determinants of myocardial oxygen demand (heart rate, contractile state, and wall tension) frequently trigger ischemia by increasing

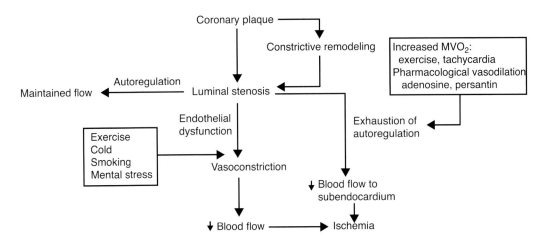

Figure 1 Schematic describing the pathophysiology of myocardial ischemia in stable coronary disease.

myocardial oxygen requirements. An increase in myocardial oxygen requirement leads to an absolute reduction in blood flow to the subendocardial region with an endo-to-epicardial flow redistribution (endo-epi steal) because of a much more limited vasodilator flow reserve in the subendocardium compared with the subepicardium. Normally the subendocardial layers of the left ventricle have 25% greater blood flow than the subepicardium because of greater systolic compressive forces and wall stress and greater level of vasodilation in the region. Because of a greater level of vasodilation at rest, the flow reserve in the subendocardium is reduced, accounting for the greater susceptibility of the subendocardium to ischemia when there is a reduction in the subendocardial driving pressure (difference between the coronary perfusion pressure and the ventricular diastolic pressure) or increase in heart rate. Normally epicardial coronary arteries serve predominantly as conduits offering little resistance to blood flow. With a progressive increase in the severity of coronary artery stenosis, the resting myocardial blood flow is maintained until the stenosis is around 90% of the diameter (Gould et al, 1974). However, peak hyperemic response (flow reserve) to brief total occlusion or in response to an arteriolar dilator stimulus such as papaverine or dipyridamole is reduced at a diameter stenosis of about 50%–60%. Maintenance of resting blood flow in the face of an increasing severity of epicardial stenosis has been attributed by some to progressive resting arteriolar dilation downstream from stenosis thereby using up the flow reserve to maintain resting flow (autoregulation). In addition to the fixed stenosis caused by atherosclerosis, passive collapse of the compliant portion of a coronary artery with an eccentric stenosis, due to a fall in upstream distending aortic pressure, can add a dynamic component to the stenosis severity thereby precipitating ischemia (Freudenberg and Lichtlen, 1981; Schwartz and Bache, 1985).

Alterations in vascular tone also add a dynamic component to the luminal stenosis in coronary artery disease. Over the last two decades, the critical role of endothelium in the modulation of vascular tone in large arteries as well as arterioles has been established (Lerman and Burnett, 1992; Harrison 1996; Furchgott and Zawadski, 1980). Several studies have shown that normal healthy endothelium triggers vasodilation in response to a variety of stimuli, such as shear stress, acetylcholine, serotonin, norepinephrine, thrombin, substance P, adenine nucleotides, and bradykinin, leading to endothelium-dependent vasodilation in both large arteries as well as in the microcirculation (Lerman and Burnett, 1992; Harrison, 1996). However, when endothelium is structurally damaged or functionally abnormal (in atherosclerotic vessels and in the presence of risk factors for atherosclerosis even without anatomic atherosclerosis), vasodilator responses to these endothelium-dependent vasodilators are attenuated, and paradoxical vasoconstriction can occur. In contrast, vasodilator responses to endothelium-independent vasodilators, such as nitroglycerin and sodium nitroprusside, are usually normal. Abnormal vasoconstrictor responses are also generally associated with abnormal vasoconstrictor responses to physiologic stimuli such as physical exercise, mental stress, cold exposure, and increased shear stress (Lerman and Burnett,

1992; Harrison, 1996; Ludmer et al, 1986; Vita et al, 1990; Yeung et al, 1991). Thus, abnormal vasoconstriction in response to physical or mental stress superimposed on a coronary stenosis may contribute to transient worsening of the severity of coronary stenosis. This effect, coupled with a reduced microvascular vasodilator function, may thus trigger myocardial ischemia during activities such as mental stress, physical exercise, and cold exposure. The normal endothelium synthesizes several vasoactive molecules that include vasodilators such as nitric oxide (NO), prostacyclin, and a hyperpolarizing factor and vasoconstrictors such as endothelin, angiotensin II, and vasoconstricting prostanoids (Palmer et al, 1987; Moncada et al, 1977; Bauersachs et al, 1994; Yanagisawa et al, 1988). Reduced vasodilator responses in atherosclerosis and in the presence of risk factors to atherosclerosis have been largely attributed to reduced production or increased inactivation of NO, one of the key vasodilator signaling molecules produced by healthy endothelium. Several studies have demonstrated that endothelium constitutively produces small amounts of NO from arginine through the action of an enzyme called NO synthase (NOS) (Lerman and Burnett, 1992; Harrison, 1996). NO rapidly diffuses into the vascular media where it increases cyclic guanosine monophosphate (GMP) levels in smooth muscle cells. Cyclic GMP serves as a substrate for cyclic GMP–dependent protein kinase, which is essential for the intracelluar calcium-lowering effects of the cyclic nucleotide leading to relaxation of the vascular smooth muscle cells. NO also has other biological effects that include reduction in endothelial adhesivity for inflammatory cells, an antiplatelet effect, and antiproliferative effect on vascular smooth muscle cells (Lerman and Burnett, 1992; Harrison, 1996). In addition to a defective NO pathway, increased endothelin production and responsiveness of vascular smooth muscle cell may also contribute to an enhanced vasoconstrictor tendency in coronary artery disease.

Several studies have demonstrated an improvement in endothelium-mediated vasodilator function with aggressive modification of risk factors accompanied by reduction in the frequency of symptomatic as well as silent myocardial ischemia (Treasure et al, 1995; Anderson et al, 1995).

PATHOPHYSIOLOGY OF ISCHEMIA AND NECROSIS IN UNSTABLE CORONARY ARTERY DISEASE (ACUTE CORONARY SYNDROMES)

Role of plaque disruption and thrombosis

It is now generally accepted that unstable angina and myocardial infarction are triggered by coronary thrombosis resulting in an abrupt increase in coronary stenosis with a resultant decrease in coronary blood flow as in unstable angina or total prolonged occlusion resulting in acute myocardial infarction (Figure 2) (Falk et al, 1995; Shah, 1998; Shah, 1997). Coronary thrombi tend to be dynamic with episodic growth, lysis, incorporation into the plaque, and downstream embolization contributing to the episodic effects on coronary blood flow. A coronary thrombus generally evolves from disruption of an atherosclerotic plaque. Disruption of an atherosclerotic plaque occurs in two main forms: (1) classic plaque rupture or plaque fissure accounting for 60%–80% of coronary thrombi; (2) plaque erosion accounting for 20%–40% of coronary thrombi (Burke et al, 1997). Plaques that rupture and produce coronary thrombi are generally large, but prior to rupture may not be severely occlusive on angiography because of outward expansion of adventitia (positive remodeling) (Falk et al, 1995; Shah, 1998). Such plaques tend to have a large necrotic lipid core with increased infiltration by macrophages, T cells, mast cells, increased neovascularity, fewer smooth muscle cells, and thinned-out fibrous caps (Shah, 1998). Plaques with these attributes have, by inference, been considered to be vulnerable plaques prior to their rupture. On the other hand, plaque erosions usually occur in plaques on a proteoglycan-rich surface without a lipid-rich core (Burke et al, 1997). The precise mechanisms that lead to either plaque rupture or plaque erosion are not well understood. It has been hypothesized that excessive extracellular matrix degradation through the release of a family of matrix-degrading enzymes (matrix-degrading metalloproteinases or MMPs and cysteine proteases such as cathepsins) as well as increased death of matrix synthesizing vascular smooth muscle cells through apoptosis may deplete the collagen framework in the fibrous cap (Shah, 1998). Depletion of collagen in the fibrous cap results in cap thinning and eventual disruption either

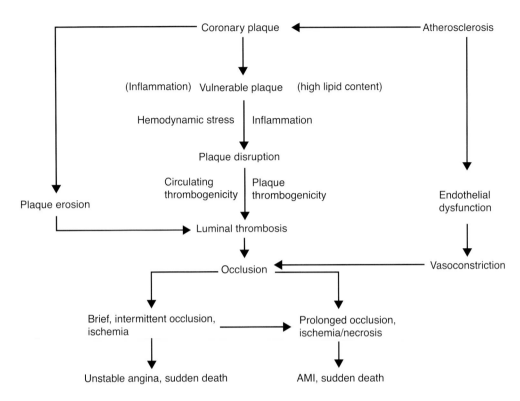

Figure 2 Schematic describing the pathophysiology of myocardial ischemia in acute and unstable coronary artery disease. AMI, acute myocardial infarction.

spontaneously or in response to hemodynamic stresses. A family of MMPs and cysteine proteases are expressed in atherosclerotic lesions where they are predominantly produced by inflammatory cells (mostly macrophages) (Shah, 1998).

Activation of inflammatory cells by various cytokines, immune mechanisms, and immunomodulatory molecules, such as CD 40, mast cell–derived proteases, oxidant stress oxidized lipids, and infectious agents such as Chlamydia pneumoniae (found in about 50% of plaques) and matrix molecules such as tenascin-c produced by macrophages in the plaque may contribute to a net increase in matrix-degrading activity by upregulation of MMPs in atherosclerotic lesions (Shah, 1998). In addition, activated inflammatory cells and toxic components of oxidized lipids in the plaque may further contribute to plaque disruption by reducing matrix content through stimulation of smooth muscle cell death by apoptosis. The magnitude and the duration of the thrombotic response following plaque disruption is likely determined by the thrombogenicity of the plaque constituents, the local rheology related to severity of stenosis and consequent shear rate, and the systemic thrombotic-antithrombotic as well as fibrinolytic-antifibrinolytic balance (Shah, 1998). Among the plaque components, the lipid core appears to be highly thrombogenic due to its high tissue factor content; tissue factor in turn is predominantly produced by the inflammatory cells (mostly the macrophages) in the plaque.

MYOCARDIAL CONSEQUENCES OF CORONARY FLOW CESSATION

When coronary blood flow falls, subendocardial ischemia occurs because of poor flow reserve and high metabolic needs. The innermost few cell layers of the endocardium remain resistant to ischemia because of direct diffusion of oxygen from cavitary blood. However, the subendocardial layers begin to show necrosis within about 20 min following cessation of blood flow. Ischemic necrosis spreads from the subendocardium towards the subepicardium in a time-dependent wave-front fashion (Reimer and Jennings, 1979; Ganz et al, 1990). This endo- to epicardial spread of necrosis is accelerated when residual blood flow is limited due to lack of collateral flow or complete and persistent coronary occlusion or when myocardial metabolic needs are high. Conversely, the spread of necrosis is slowed or halted in the presence of residual flow through incomplete or intermittent coronary occlusion or immediate recruitment of well-developed collaterals. The time-dependent evolution of myocardial necrosis following coronary artery occlusion provides a narrow window of opportunity during which successful reperfusion can abort the wave-front of necrosis thereby limiting infarct size, attenuating myocardial dysfunction, and improving clinical outcome in patients with acute myocardial infarction.

STUNNING, HIBERNATION, AND ISCHEMIC PRECONDITIONING

Myocardial stunning refers to systolic and diastolic myocardial dysfunction that persists beyond the duration of ischemia (Marban, 1991). This prolonged myocardial dysfunction is followed by gradual recovery over hours, days, or weeks. Despite lack of contractile function at rest, the myocardium remains responsive to inotropic stimulation. The intensity of ischemia and the duration of ischemia appear to be the major determinants of the degree of postischemic reversible dysfunction. Clinically, myocardial stunning is often seen during unstable angina due to intermittent episodes of ischemia at rest, acute myocardial infarction followed by spontaneous or therapeutic reperfusion, and following ischemic cardiac arrest during cardiopulmonary bypass. The precise metabolic and biochemical basis for myocardial stunning is poorly understood. Chronic reduction in myocardial perfusion due to severe coronary stenoses or collateralized total occlusion may also lead to depressed contractile function and adaptive changes in myocardial metabolism resulting in a state of myocardial "hibernation" with noncontractile but viable myocardium (Marban, 1991). Proof of viability is evident when these nonfunctional myocardial segments recover their contractile function following restoration of blood flow through revascularization. From a clinical standpoint, patients with coronary artery disease with severely depressed ventricular function and chronic congestive heart failure may benefit symptomatically and with an improved prognosis with revascularization when noninvasive imaging studies provide evidence of viability in noncontractile myocardial segments (Di Carli et al, 1998).

Brief periods of coronary occlusion followed by reperfusion prior to a more prolonged sustained coronary artery occlusion lasting 1.5–3 h result in a substantive reduction in infarct size independent of collateral flow. These observations have led to the concept of ischemic preconditioning. The precise biochemical mediators of this interesting phenomenon are not fully understood. Potential mediators include activation of an energy-sparing ATP-activated potassium channel, slowing of glycolysis with attenuation of intracellular acidosis, and molecular adaptation with induction of heat shock protein (Chen et al, 1995; Gross and Auchampach, 1992). In humans, observations of a reduced infarct size, better preserved ventricular function, and lower mortality of Q-wave acute myocardial infarction (AMI) patients in whom the AMI was preceded by preinfarction angina (a clinical surrogate for brief periods of ischemia) compared with those without antecedent preinfarction angina, is considered a potential example of ischemic preconditioning (Anzai et al, 1995).

PROTECTIVE ROLE OF CORONARY COLLATERALS

Collaterals are vascular channels that connect epicardial coronary arteries providing alternate sources of blood flow distal to a coronary artery obstruction. These interconnecting vascular channels, which are present in normal hearts, range in diameter from 20–200 μm and their density varies greatly among different individuals and species (Kanazawa, 1994). These collateral channels, although anatomically present, remain functionally closed under normal circumstances because of a lack of a pressure gradient between the donor and recipient arteries. However, when a coronary artery stenosis and obstruction are imposed, the poststenotic or postobstructive pressure decline creates an immediate gradient for flow from the high-pressure donor vessel to the low-pressure recipient vessel opening up the collateral channels. Following opening, the thin-walled collateral channels undergo several anatomic changes that transform them into three-layer structures resembling epicardial coronary arteries and ultimately resulting in nearly a 10-fold increase in luminal diameter. Endogenous endothelium–derived NO and prostacyclin have been shown to regulate collateral blood flow.

Coronary collaterals clearly play a protective role in coronary artery disease. Mature collaterals can maintain normal blood flow to poststenotic or postocclusive segments at rest and during moderate exercise, but with maximal exercise or pharmacological vasodilation collateral flow may not be sufficient to preclude the development of subendocardial ischemia. Collaterals can significantly attenuate the severity of ischemia related to critical coronary artery obstruction, reduce the extent of myocardial necrosis and contractile dysfunction following acute coronary occlusion, maintain myocardium in a viable but noncontractile state (hibernating myocardium) following coronary occlusion, and in some cases completely prevent the development of myocardial infarction and ventricular dysfunction in the face of total coronary artery occlusion. In humans, angiographic evidence of functional collaterals are rarely observed until a diameter coronary stenosis of greater than 70%. This highlights the importance of a pressure gradient for the opening up of preexisting collateral channels. A number of studies have examined the effects of chronic exercise on coronary collateral development in animals and humans but the overall results have not been encouraging. In recent years, local or systemic administration of angiogenic growth factors, such as fibroblast growth factor (FGF) and vascular endothelial growth factor (VEGF), using either recombinant forms of these proteins, naked DNA encoding these proteins, or viral vectors carrying the DNA encoding these proteins, has been tested in experimental models of limb and cardiac ischemia and shown to promote collateral and neovascular growth (Isner et al, 1995).

Human studies with these angiogenic factors are currently ongoing for peripheral and coronary artery disease.

SUMMARY

Myocardial ischemia results from a dynamic interplay between several pathophysiologic processes that determine coronary blood flow and myocardial oxygen and energy needs. A fixed coronary stenosis due to buildup of an atherosclerotic plaque reduces coronary flow reserve whereas vasoconstriction in the coronary lesion as well as impaired vasodilator capacity of the microcirculation, due to endothelial dysfunction, contribute a dynamic component. Together these factors lead to episodic coronary flow reduction and endo- to epicardial flow redistribution that leads to myocardial ischemia. In unstable coronary syndromes, a coronary thrombus superimposed on a disrupted plaque creates yet another mechanism for additional dynamic coronary obstruction which plays a critical role in mediating episodic flow reductions and myocardial ischemia. In addition to episodic chronic or acute myocardial ischemia, a chronic state of myocardial ischemia (hibernation) also exists that can contribute to ventricular dysfunction and congestive heart failure. Finally, repetitive brief episodes of ischemia may attenuate the extent of necrosis after a subsequent total and sustained coronary occlusion through the phenomenon of ischemic preconditioning.

CLINICAL IMPLICATIONS

An improved understanding of the role of not only the fixed coronary stenosis due to atherosclerosis but also the role of endothelial dysfunction, vasoconstriction, and plaque disruption with thrombosis has led to improved therapeutic options for alleviation of myocardial ischemia.

CHAPTER 10

EFFICACY OF IVABRADINE IN STABLE ANGINA

KIM FOX

INTRODUCTION

Stable angina is a common clinical syndrome that often seriously limits patients' everyday activities. Anginal symptoms occur as a result of myocardial ischemia due to an imbalance between myocardial perfusion and the demands of the myocardium. A reduction in heart rate improves endocardial blood supply and decreases myocardial oxygen demand. Agents that reduce the heart rate would, therefore, be predicted to exert a beneficial effect on both elements of this imbalance.

A new class of selective heart rate–lowering agents has been developed that act on the sinoatrial node of the heart by inhibiting the inward hyperpolarization-activated I_f current, which is probably the most important pacemaker current of the sinoatrial node (DiFrancesco 1986, 1991; Irisawa et al, 1993). Ivabradine (Procoralan, Servier) is a specific inhibitor of I_f, which selectively blocks the pacemaker current I_f in a use-dependent manner (Bois et al, 1996, Bucchi et al, 2002). Ivabradine has produced a reduction in both resting and exercise heart rate in animals (Thollon et al, 1994; Gardiner et al, 1995; Simon et al, 1995) and healthy human volunteers (Ragueneau et al, 1998). This dose-ranging study assessed the efficacy, safety, and tolerance of different doses of ivabradine in the treatment of stable angina pectoris (Borer et al, 2003).

METHODS

This multicenter, late phase 2 study started with a 2 to 7-day wash-out period (according to the half-life of prior antianginal medication), followed by a 1-week, single-blind placebo run-in period to evaluate the stability of patients' exercise tolerance test (ETT) performance and compliance with the protocol. Then, during a double-blind, placebo-controlled 2-week period, patients were randomized to one of three doses of ivabradine (2.5, 5, or 10 mg) or placebo, twice daily (bid). Treatment was assigned (by random permutation blocks) to patients according to the chronological order of inclusion within each center. Following the double-blind period, patients voluntarily took part in an open-label extension period in which ivabradine was given 10 mg bid for 2 or 3 months to evaluate safety and maintenance of efficacy. Finally, during a 1-week double-blind, randomized withdrawal period, patients received ivabradine 10 mg or placebo bid to confirm the persistence of efficacy and evaluate disease evolution following withdrawal of treatment.

All patients provided written, informed consent prior to selection. The study was conducted in accordance with the Declaration of Helsinki (1964) as revised in Hong Kong (1989); the protocol was approved by an independent ethics committee in each participating country.

Patients (male, or female of non–child-bearing potential) aged 18 years or older with a history of chronic stable angina for at least 3 months (triggered by physical activity and relieved by rest or nitroglycerine) were eligible for inclusion. At selection (D–7) and inclusion (D0), patients were required to have a positive and stable ETT. A positive ETT was characterized by the occurrence of both limiting angina and an ST-segment depression of at least 1 mm compared with the resting ECG. Stability of ETT performance from D–7 to D0 was evaluated by time to 1-mm ST-segment depression, and could differ by no more than 20% or 1 min.

Other inclusion criteria were: documented coronary artery disease (coronary angiography showing 50% stenosis in the proximal two-thirds of at least one major coronary artery, or (for males) be on a waiting list for coronary angiography and have a previous positive exercise thallium scan, or previous dipyramidole, dobutamine, or exercise echocardiography test showing a hypokinetic or akinetic segment during exercise); or typical angina pain more than 6 months after a coronary angioplasty or more than

3 months following a coronary artery bypass graft (CABG); or previous myocardial infarction 3 or more months prior to randomization; compliance of at least 75% with placebo during the run-in.

Exclusion criteria included: coronary angioplasty within the previous 6 months; significant valvular disease; atrial fibrillation, flutter or use of a pacemaker; 2nd and 3rd degree atrioventricular block, or resting bradycardia (< 50 beats per minute), or sick sinus syndrome; unstable, microvascular or Prinzmetal angina; recent acute myocardial infarction or coronary bypass surgery within the previous 3 months; inability to perform ETT.

Primary efficacy criteria were the changes in time to 1-mm ST-segment depression (horizontal or down-sloping for more than 0.08 s after the J point) and time to limiting angina during ETT at the trough of drug activity (12 h postdose). Secondary efficacy criteria included: changes over time in other ETT criteria at the trough of drug activity; changes in ETT criteria at the peak of drug activity (4 h postdose); angina attack frequency as recorded in patients' diaries.

Safety was assessed by adverse events, cardiovascular events (blood pressure during ETT, ECG at rest, 24-h Holter monitoring in a subset of 75 patients equally distributed between the treatment groups), vital signs, and laboratory tests.

Statistical methods

Pretreatment between-group comparability and between-group comparisons of primary and secondary efficacy criteria were conducted using the Kruskal-Wallis test and a one-way analysis of variance. The active groups were compared with placebo using the two-tailed Dunnett's test and the equivalent nonparametric approach, in the case of a significant group effect. In the case of a significant treatment effect, with at least one ivabradine dose different from placebo, the dose–effect relationship was studied using linear regression.

Efficacy analyses were conducted in the per-protocol (PP) population and intention-to-treat (ITT) populations. The PP population comprised patients completing the study period without major protocol violations, and having trough ETT results at the end of the study period with an evaluable time to 1-mm ST-segment depression at baseline. The safety population comprised all randomized patients receiving at least one treatment dose. Safety variables were analyzed using descriptive statistics. Unless otherwise indicated, data are presented as means ± standard deviations. Quoted P values are from parametric analyses; $P < 0.05$ was considered to be significant.

Results

Of 529 patients screened, 400 were included in the trial; ineligibility was primarily due to a negative ETT at the selection visit ($n = 100$). A total of 360 patients were randomized to receive ivabradine during the double-blind, placebo-controlled period; 40 selected patients were not randomized, 23 because of a negative ETT at D0. Baseline characteristics of randomized patients are shown in Table 1; there were no clinically relevant differences in baseline characteristics between the randomized ($n = 360$) and PP ($n = 257$) populations. Unless stated otherwise, results are presented for the PP population.

Efficacy

Heart rate
Ivabradine produced a significant dose-dependent reduction in both resting and maximal heart rate at both the trough and peak of drug activity during the double-blind period (Figure 1). All three ivabradine dose levels were significantly different from placebo for both parameters at both timepoints of drug activity.

Time to 1-mm ST-segment depression and limiting angina
Ivabradine, at doses of 5 and 10 mg bid, produced a significant increase, compared with placebo, in time to 1-mm ST-segment depression during ETT at both trough and peak of drug activity (Figure 2a); there

TABLE 1. Baseline characteristics of the randomized population in the double-blind, dose-ranging period. Data are given as means ± standard deviations, except where indicated.

	RANDOMIZED POPULATION ($n = 360$)	
Age (years)	58.5 ± 9.2	
Gender (male/female)	323/37	
Weight (kg)	79.0 ± 11.2	
Blood pressure (supine) (mmHg)		
Systolic	133.7 ± 16.3	
Diastolic	81.3 ± 8.2	
Supine heart rate (bpm)	69.7 ± 10.3	
Coronary artery disease duration (months)	68.1 ± 63.9	
Mean frequency of angina attacks (per week)	5.3 ± 7.9	
Mean consumption of short-acting nitrates (units/week)	3.4 ± 7.6	
History of:		DELAY (MONTHS)
Myocardial infarction; n [%]	218 [60.6]	66 ± 65
Coronary artery bypass graft; n [%]	59 [16.4]	74 ± 65
Percutaneous transluminal coronary angioplasty; n [%]	66 [18.3]	37 ± 34

was a significant dose–effect relationship ($P = 0.005$). Ivabradine also increased the time to limiting angina (Figure 2b) and time to angina onset (Table 2); for both parameters, pairwise comparisons with placebo reached significance for the 10 mg ivabradine group at both trough and peak drug activity and for the 5 mg group only at peak drug activity. Ivabradine also produced significant, dose-dependent reductions in rate pressure product (heart rate × systolic blood pressure), both at rest and at the peak of exercise (Table 2). The magnitude of changes in these ergometric criteria was greater at the peak of drug activity than at the trough of drug activity.

In the ITT population, the pattern of changes in the double-blind, placebo-controlled period was similar to that in the PP population, except that changes in time to limiting angina at the trough of drug activity did not achieve statistical significance ($P = 0.058$; data not shown).

In the open-label extension period, the improvements in time to 1-mm ST-segment depression produced by ivabradine in the double-blind period were fully maintained (Figure 3), and patients switching from placebo to ivabradine showed a dramatic improvement. The time to limiting angina followed a similar pattern (data not shown). During the open-label extension period, time to 1-mm ST-segment depression improved by more than 1 min for the patient population as a whole ($P < 0.001$ for this change and the change in the time to limiting angina in both the PP and ITT populations).

Withdrawal period

Patients continuing on ivabradine treatment during the double-blind withdrawal period showed maintained improvements in ETT parameters, such as resting heart rate, time to 1-mm ST-segment depression, and time to limiting angina (Figure 4; Table 3). In contrast, patients switching to placebo showed significant deteriorations in all major ETT parameters measured with no rebound phenomena on treatment withdrawal.

Angina attacks

Ivabradine reduced both the number of angina attacks and consumption of short-acting nitrates during the double-blind period, but the changes did not reach statistical significance. During the open-label extension period, ivabradine reduced the mean number of angina attacks/week from 4.14 ± 5.59 at baseline to 0.95 ± 2.24 ($P < 0.001$) and the consumption of short-acting nitrates from a mean of 2.28 ± 3.74 units/week to 0.50 ± 1.14 units/week ($P < 0.001$). During the withdrawal period, the angina attack frequency was unchanged in patients continuing with ivabradine but increased (by 0.74 ± 1.95 attacks/week) in those switching to placebo, although the between-group difference was not significant ($P = 0.067$).

(a)

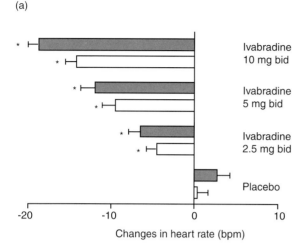

(b)

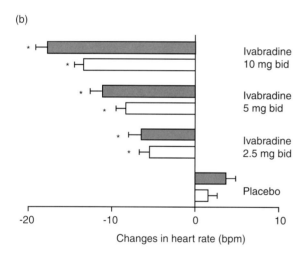

FIGURE 1. (a) Changes in heart rate at rest (pre-exercise), and **(b)** changes in maximal heart rate during ETT, at trough (white bars) and peak (grey bars) of drug activity. Data are given as mean ± SEM; *$P < 0.05$ versus placebo. Modified with permission from Borer et al, 2003.

Safety

During the double-blind, multidose period, the incidence of adverse events was low and generally similar in all of the ivabradine and placebo groups. However, the incidence of visual symptoms was higher in the ivabradine groups (2.5 mg, $n = 1$; 5 mg, $n = 1$, 10 mg, $n = 13$) than in the placebo group ($n = 0$). During the open-label extension period, a similar pattern of adverse events was noted, with 31 patients reporting visual symptoms, which were mild in 29 patients. During the withdrawal period, visual symptoms were reported by one patient. Only three patients withdrew (all voluntarily and not at the investigators' insistence because of safety concerns) from the study due to visual symptoms. There were no serious cardiac events reported following treatment withdrawal, suggesting the absence of rebound phenomena.

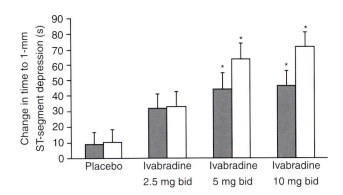

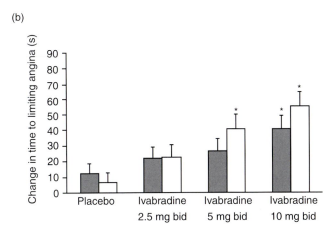

FIGURE 2. (a) Changes in time to 1-mm ST-segment depression, and (b) changes in time to limiting angina, at trough (grey bars) and peak (white bars) of drug activity. Data are given as means ± SEM; *$P < 0.05$ vs placebo.

DISCUSSION

There is mounting evidence to indicate that a high heart rate is associated with increased cardiovascular morbidity and mortality (Fujiura et al, 2001; Kristal-Boneh et al, 2000; Palatini and Julius 1999; Seccareccia et al, 2001). In the current study in patients with stable angina pectoris, the novel selective and specific I_f inhibitor ivabradine was an effective heart rate–lowering agent. Ivabradine produced significant, dose-dependent reductions in heart rate, both at rest and at the peak of exercise at the peak and trough of drug activity. The magnitude of heart rate lowering achieved with ivabradine 10 mg bid in angina patients was similar to that reported with a similar dose in healthy volunteers (Ragueneau et al, 1998).

Ivabradine doses of 5 and 10 mg bid were also associated with significant improvements in ergometric criteria during ETT, such as time to reach 1-mm ST-segment depression and time to limiting angina. These improvements were maintained throughout the entire trial duration by those patients receiving ivabradine, but all major ETT criteria significantly deteriorated in patients switched to placebo during the withdrawal period.

The efficacy of ivabradine in the current study is comparable to that achieved historically with β-blockers in patients with angina. β-Blockers reduce heart rate and are recommended as initial treatment in stable angina in the absence of contraindications (Fihn et al, 2001), particularly in post–myocardial

TABLE 2. Changes in time to angina onset and rate pressure product (RPP) measured at the trough and peak of drug activity during the double-blind, dose-ranging period[a] – per-protocol population.

PARAMETER	IVABRADINE 2.5 MG BID (n = 64)	IVABRADINE 5 MG BID (n = 59)	IVABRADINE 10 MG BID (n = 66)	PLACEBO (n = 68)	BETWEEN-GROUP P VALUE
Trough					
Time to angina onset (s)	37.6 ± 57.7	38.8 ± 81.7	69.4 ± 74.8*	24.7 ± 64.2	0.003
RPP at rest (bpm.mmHg)	–509 ± 1697	–1366 ± 1950*	–1909 ± 1688*	178 ± 2218	< 0.001
RPP at peak of exercise (bpm.mmHg)	–737 ± 2950	–1142 ± 3354*	–1543 ± 3526*	266 ± 3074	0.011
Peak					
Time to angina onset (s)	44.9 ± 69.0	72.1 ± 83.1*	94.9 ± 88.5*	28.9 ± 66.5	< 0.001
RPP at rest (bpm.mmHg)	–740 ± 1696*	–1740 ± 2059*	–2621 ± 1672*	167 ± 1952	< 0.001
RPP at peak of exercise (bpm.mmHg)	–931 ± 3730*	–1490 ± 3774*	–2148 ± 3057*	765 ± 3389	< 0.001

[a] Expressed as value on D14 *minus* value on D0; mean ± standard deviation
*Significantly different from placebo in pairwise comparison.

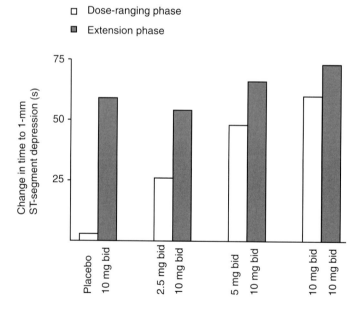

FIGURE 3. Changes in time to 1-mm ST-segment depression in ETT, measured at the trough of drug activity, in patients continuing in the open-label extension period (D14–D104), by treatment group during the double-blind dose-ranging period (D0–D14). All patients received ivabradine 10 mg bid during the open-label extension period. Ivabradine dosages during the first randomized treatment were 2.5 mg bid; 5 mg bid; 10 mg bid; and placebo. For approximately 10% of patients, the extension period ended after 2 months; these data are shown pooled with those ending the extension period after 3 months.

infarction patients (Management of stable angina pectoris, 1997; Gibbons et al, 1999). However, β-blockers also reduce myocardial contractility and can cause paradoxical vasoconstriction of large epicardial arteries in animals (Berdeaux et al, 1991; Simon et al, 1995) and humans (Bortone et al, 1990). β-Blockers may be contraindicated in a relatively high proportion of patients. Traditional contraindications include

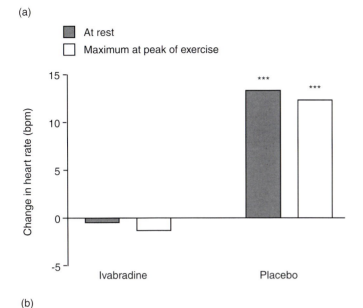

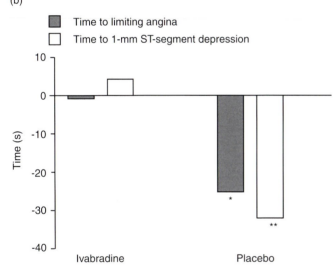

FIGURE 4. (a) Changes in heart rate during the randomized withdrawal period, measured at trough of drug activity. (b) Changes in time to limiting angina and 1-mm ST-segment depression during the randomized withdrawal period, measured at trough of drug activity. Values expressed as value at end of withdrawal period minus value at end of open-label extension period. *$P = 0.018$; **$P = 0.003$; ***$P < 0.001$ versus placebo.

obstructive airway disease (Boskabady and Snashall, 2000; Tattersfield, 1991), and also peripheral vascular disease (Lewis and Lofthouse, 1993), which often coexists with coronary artery disease. Patients with hypotension or higher than first-degree heart block are also not considered appropriate candidates for β-blockade (Ramahi, 2000). β-Blockers may also have adverse effects on lipid and carbohydrate metabolism (Krone and Nagele, 1988; Pollare et al, 1989; Skarfors et al, 1989; Lithell et al, 1992; Hakamaki and Lehtonen, 1997; Reneland et al, 2000). Moreover, the need for more selective heart rate–lowering agents was further underlined by a primary care study of chronic stable angina patients which concluded that anginal symptoms were often poorly controlled, even though almost two thirds of patients were on more than one cardiovascular drug (Pepine et al, 1994).

Ivabradine belongs to a new class of specific heart rate–lowering agents. It is a selective and specific inhibitor of the hyperpolarization-activated inward I_f current, one of the most important currents in pacemaking in the sinoatrial node (DiFrancesco, 1991). In animal studies, ivabradine had little action on other cardiac ionic currents or cardiac action potential shape (Thollon et al, 1994; Bois et al, 1996) and

TABLE 3. Changes in time to angina onset, rate pressure product (RPP) at rest and at peak of exercise, measured at the trough of drug activity, during the randomized withdrawal period[a] – per-protocol population.

PARAMETER	IVABRADINE 10 MG BID (n = 59)	PLACEBO (n = 65)	BETWEEN-GROUP P VALUE
Time to angina onset (s)	2.1 ± 59.1	−36.05 ± 76.7	0.002
RPP at rest (bpm.mmHg)	−26 ± 1207	1487 ± 1628	< 0.001
RPP at peak of exercise (bpm.mmHg)	−180 ± 3195	1813 ± 3331	< 0.001

[a] Expressed as value at end of withdrawal period *minus* value at end of open-label extension period; mean ± standard deviation.

did not significantly affect myocardial contractility (Simon et al, 1995; Bel et al, 1998). Thus, direct and specific inhibition of I_f channels may allow heart rate reduction with minimal change to other myocardial properties.

In the current study, ivabradine was associated with excellent cardiovascular tolerability. The only treatment-related adverse events were visual symptoms associated with the 10 mg bid dose. Such symptoms were not unexpected, having previously occurred in a study in healthy volunteers (Ragueneau et al, 1998). Such visual symptoms tend to be of mild to moderate intensity and to resolve spontaneously without sequelae, and may be linked to the presence of channels in the retina that are similar to I_f channels (Kaneko and Tachibana, 1985; Demontis et al. 1999; Satoh and Yamada, 2000). Importantly, there was no 'rebound' phenomenon on withdrawal of ivabradine, unlike the rebound increase in ischemic activity that occurs after abrupt withdrawal of β-blockade in patients with chronic stable angina (e.g. Egstrup, 1988).

In conclusion, in this first large-scale clinical trial in patients with stable angina pectoris, ivabradine produced dose-dependent reductions in resting and exercise heart rates and displayed antianginal and/or anti-ischemic efficacy at doses of 5 and 10 mg bid. Ivabradine showed no evidence of rebound phenomenon or pharmacological tolerance, and was associated with good clinical acceptability, tolerability, and safety. The specific heart rate–lowering activity of ivabradine may offer an effective and safe alternative to current medical treatment options in stable angina.

ACKNOWLEDGMENTS

European Ivabradine Late Phase 2 Investigators Group:
Belgium: G. Heyndrickx, Aalst; M. Vrolix, Genk.
Czech Republic: J. Bultas, Praha; J. Janousek, Beroun; O. Jerabek, Zdabor; V. Stanek, Praha; J. Vrany, Praha.
France: P. Delelis, Lambersart; R. Dimitriou, Voiron; S. Elhadad, Lagny-sur-Marne; K. Khalife, Metz; J.-C. Louchart, Bethune; E. Page, Grenoble.
Germany: H. Becker, Hanau; U. Biermann, Altenkirchen; L. Hopf, Frankfurt; M. Keck, Bad Munster; G. Kober, Bad Nauheim; G. Rettig Sturmer, Sulzbach; E. Von Czako, Saarbrucken.
Hungary: R. De Chatel, Budapest; A. Janosi, Budapest; L. Matos, Budapest; I. Préda, Budapest; K. Toth, Pecs.
Poland: L. Giec, Katowice; M. Krzeminska Pakula, Lodz; J. Kuch, Warsaw; W. Ruzyllo, Warsaw; A. Rynkiewicz, Gdansk; Z. Sadowski, Warsaw.
Russian Federation: I. Chazov, Moscow; A. Golikov, Moscow; V. Makolkin, Moscow; V. Metelitsa, Moscow.
Spain: J. Bardaji, Cuenca; J. Bruguera, Barcelona; J. Cruz Fernandez, Seville; C. Fernandez Palomeque, Palma de Mallorca; J. Gonzalez Juanatey, Santiago de Compostela; C. Macaya, Madrid; C. Pagola, Jaen; L. Rodriguez Padial, Toledo.
United Kingdom: P. Bennett, Bath; J. Davies, Newport; K. Fox, London; D. Lindsay, Gloucester; W. Littler, Birmingham; B. Silke, Belfast; S. Singh, Birmingham; J. Stephens, Romford; G. Sutton, Uxbridge.

CHAPTER 11

CLINICAL INTEREST OF HEART RATE REDUCTION IN HEART FAILURE

Sergio Chierchia and Antonio Zingarelli

INTRODUCTION

Myocardial contraction is biochemically influenced by the functional integrity of the actomyosin system and by the intracellular concentration of calcium ions (Ca^{++}) that is maintained by the efficiency of the sarcolemmal membrane and sarcoplasmic reticulum. The former, by means of voltage-dependent and receptor-operated Ca^{++} channels and by the sarcolemmal Ca^{++}-ATPase pump, regulates the inflow and outflow of cellular calcium; the latter causes its release and storage through the activity of a series of specific proteins such as calmodulin, phospholamban, and sarcoplasmic Ca^{++}-ATPase. The interaction between the actomyosin system and intracellular calcium is regulated by the troponin–tropomyosin complex. When the calcium concentration rises within the cell during depolarization, the troponin C subunit binds calcium, inhibits the binding of the troponin I subunit to actin, and triggers the interaction between actin and myosin.

Under physiological conditions, myocardial contraction depends on four fundamental factors, reciprocally correlated:
1. Preload, governed by the Frank-Starling's law that links the force of contraction to the resting length of myocardial fibers. This is determined by the initial load that precedes contraction and is influenced by ventricular compliance.
2. Afterload, defined as the tension or stress acting on myocardial fibers when shortening begins: in the intact organism, afterload is determined by aortic impedance and systemic arterial resistance as well as blood volume and viscosity.
3. Contractility, a fundamental intrinsic property of cardiac muscle, defined as the velocity and extent of myocardial fiber shortening at a determined instantaneous load.
4. Frequency of contraction, expressed *in vivo* by the heart rate.

Clinically, myocardial function is mainly expressed by the cardiac output, a variable that depends on two physiological determinants, heart rate and stroke volume. Increase or preservation of adequate cardiac output may be obtained by varying one or both of these variables.

Any condition that leads to "pump" dysfunction activates both of these mechanisms through a number of neural and neurohumoral pathways in an attempt to maintain adequate perfusion pressure to peripheral organs, particularly brain and kidneys.

As a result, patients with heart failure frequently present with compensatory tachycardia, which may be sufficient to produce an adequate cardiac output if ventricular function is preserved and stroke volume is reduced because of impaired venous return. However, tachycardia may no longer be compensatory but even further deteriorate the performance of the failing heart with systolic or diastolic dysfunction. In a recent trial conducted in more than 2700 outpatients with heart failure, heart rate greater than 100 beats per minute seemed to contribute to predicting the short-term risk of cardiac decompensation with an incremental risk of 61% (Opasich et al, 2001).

Besides, in the advanced chronic phase, adrenergic hyperactivity and persistently elevated levels of plasma cathecholamines may further compromise myocardial dysfunction by causing progressive abnormalities in signal transduction, resulting in downregulation of myocardial β-adrenergic receptor density and lower myocardial receptor density (Bristow et al, 1982; Fowler et al, 1986).

For these and for a number of other reasons, reducing the heart rate has always been regarded as a desirable therapeutic target in the failing heart. Indeed, a longer diastole favors ventricular filling and increases stroke volume. It prolongs coronary perfusion time and decreases myocardial oxygen requirements.

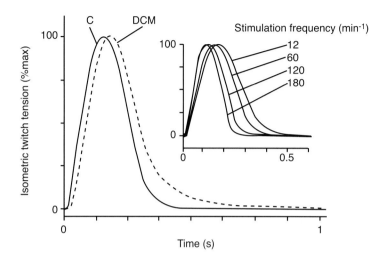

FIGURE 1. Isometric myograms from human ventricular myocardial strips at constant stimulation: comparison of nonfailing control myocardium (C) vs dilated cardiomyopathy (DCM). Inner square: twitches of normal myocardium at various stimulation frequency. Reproduced with permission from Mulieri et al, 1992.

In the past, lowering of the heart rate was attempted by digitalis or β-blockers. However, the effect of cardiac glycosides on sinus rate is minimal and the use of β-blockers may be precluded by their negative inotropic effects or other adverse reactions. Similarly, the non-dihydropyridine calcium blockers are contraindicated, because their negative effects on contractility may prove deleterious. For these reasons a number of investigators have regarded with much interest the development of new agents whose sole pharmacological effect is the reduction of the sinus node repolarization rate.

In this review, we will discuss some of the mechanisms that link heart rate to contractile function, in the normal and failing heart. We will briefly review the results obtained with traditional agents and outline the pharmacological characteristics and potential clinical applications of sinus node inhibitors.

HEART RATE AND MYOCARDIAL CONTRACTION

The physiological relationship between heart rate and myocardial contraction is described by the well-known "force-frequency relation" (Bodwitch effect, "treppe phenomenon" or staircase effect) where any increase in heart rate also increases the rate of force development as well as the developed force, shortens the time to peak tension, and accelerates relaxation (Figure 1).

However, the failing heart behaves in a totally different manner: Mulieri et al (1992) studied *in vitro* myocardial fiber properties of failing and nonfailing hearts, obtained, respectively, from explanted organs of patients with idiopathic dilated cardiomyopathy undergoing cardiac transplantation and from microbiopsy of normal myocardium performed immediately after cardiac arrest during coronary bypass surgery.

They examined the isometric twitch tension over a range of stimulation rates from 12 to 240/min. In the failing heart, peak tension was depressed by 48% at a stimulation rate of 72/min and by 80% at 174/min. Although peak twitch tensions are similar in failing and nonfailing myocardial strips in the low frequency range (12 to 40/min), this does not hold at higher stimulation frequencies. In the nonfailing myocardium, increasing the stimulation frequency from 60 to 150/min causes a doubling of twitch tension and 2.6-fold increases in peak rates of twitch tension rise and fall. In the failing myocardium, this frequency-dependent potentiation is absent or greatly attenuated. At a contraction frequency of 120/min the amplitude and rate of twitch tension are only one third of the values generated by the nonfailing myocardium (Figure 2).

Many clinical studies conducted in patients with dilated cardiomyopathy during atrial pacing have confirmed these experimental findings: no increases in the peak rate of left ventricular pressure rise were observed by Feldman et al (1988). By evaluating hemodynamic parameters in dilated cardiomyopathy during right ventricular pacing, Hasenfuss et al (1994) demonstrated a 15% reduction in cardiac output

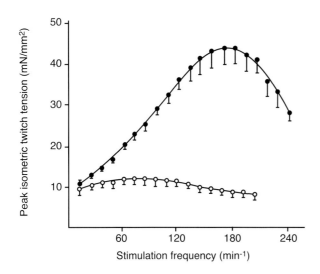

FIGURE 2. Relation of peak isometric twich tension and stimulation frequency in isolated preparations of nonfailing myocardium (○) and dilated cardiomyopathy (●). Reproduced with permission from Mulieri et al, 1992.

by increasing heart rate from 84 to 140 beats/min. The stroke volume was already reduced with a heart rate increase from 84 to 100 beats/min. Left ventricular end-diastolic volume did not decrease with increasing heart rate, indicating that the reduction in stroke volume was not due to decreased preload, but resulted from impaired ejection fraction and decreased contractility (Figures 3a,b,c).

The systolic alterations observed in the failing heart may be secondary to altered Ca^{++} homeostasis, with suboptimal intracellular concentrations available to the actomyosin complex. Furthermore, reduced Ca^{++} reuptake from the sarcoplasmic reticulum which affects diastolic relaxation can be further impaired by increasing heart rate (Gwathmey et al, 1987, 1990). Under physiological conditions, the increases in heart rate obtained by electrical pacing or β-adrenergic stimulation cause a cyclic adenosine monophosphate (cAMP)–dependent Ca^{++} influx by opening voltage-dependent and receptor-operated sarcolemmal channels, respectively, and increase contraction. However, many studies conducted in myocardial fibers from failing hearts showed sarcolemmal Ca^{++} channel dysfunction as well as altered storage of intracellular Ca^{++}. This was especially true in the sarcoplasmic reticulum where phospholamban regulates a magnesium ATP-dependent enzyme ($SR-Ca^{++}-ATPase$): the lower increase in twitch tension of failing fibers is associated with lower $SR-Ca^{++}-ATPase$ synthesis (Mercadier et al, 1990).

HEART RATE AND THE AUTONOMIC NERVOUS SYSTEM

The importance of heart rate as a risk factor for cardiovascular disease is well known: high resting heart rates are prospectively related to the development of atherosclerosis and cardiovascular events. This relationship is independent of other major risk factors for atherosclerosis and is observed in the general population, in elderly people, in hypertensive cohorts, and in patients with myocardial infarction or heart failure. The clustering of several risk factors in individuals with faster heart rates may explain why cardiovascular morbidity is higher in individuals with tachycardia. Sympathetic overactivity seems to be responsible for both the increases in heart rate and blood pressure and accounts for a number of metabolic abnormalities. Elevated heart rate can also exert a direct atherogenic action on the arterial system through increased wall stress.

An imbalance between sympathetic and parasympathetic afferents has been shown in patients with congestive heart failure (CHF) (Floras, 1993), which is explained by the activation of several autonomic reflexes, originating from the carotid sinus and the cardiopulmonary area.

Reduction in mean arterial pressure stems from arterial baroreceptor dysfunction, which results in altered capacity for stimulating vagal tone and inhibiting sympathetic activity.

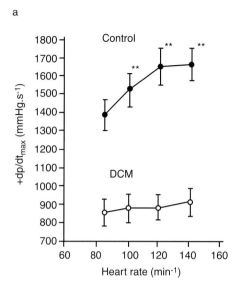

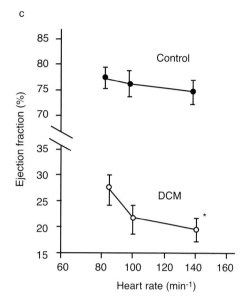

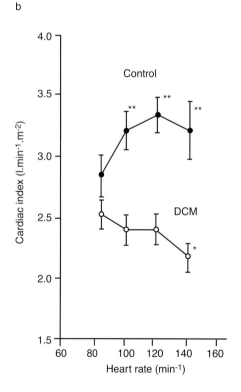

Figure 3. Influence of heart rate on, respectively, the maximum rate of left ventricular pressure development (dp/dt max) (a), cardiac index (b), and ejection fraction (c) in normal subjects (control) and in patients with dilated cardiomyopathy (DCM) (from Hasenfuss et al, 1994). *$P < 0.05$ vs lowest pacing rate; **$P < 0.01$ vs lowest pacing rate

Moreover, cardiopulmonary stretch receptors that react to changes in plasma volume are also affected and their capacity for inhibiting sympathetic activation is reduced. With acute hypotension, sympathetic hyperactivity causes arterial and venous vasoconstriction and increases heart rate, in an attempt to maintain an adequate cardiac output. In the chronic situation, heart rate is tonically increased and beat-to-beat heart rate variability (HRV), an index of sympathovagal balance, is reduced. Many studies based on spectral analysis of HRV have assessed several frequency-domain parameters and have confirmed that the low-frequency component (specific for sympathetic activity) is enhanced, and the high-frequency component (specific for parasympathetic activity) is reduced. The prognostic and independent value of time-domain HRV indices identifying patients at high risk of sudden death or progressive heart failure is now well established (Nolan et al, 1992, 1998; Tuininga et al, 1994; Bonaduce et al, 1999).

Interestingly, postural changes may also affect neuroautonomic activity in patients with CHF. For example, Fujita et al (2000) demonstrated that the right lateral decubitus, the preferred recumbent sleeping position in such patients, correlates with a very low LF/HF ratio. Indeed, when recumbent in the right lateral position, patients exhibit lower levels of plasma norepinephrine, suggesting that the preferred decubitus position acts as a self-protective mechanism attenuating sympathetic overactivity.

HEART RATE AND PHARMACOLOGICAL MODULATORS

Heart rate correlates with the depolarization frequency of specific pacemaking cells localized throughout the activation-conduction system and mostly concentrated in the sinoatrial node where their firing rate is the highest. Electrophysiologically, the action potentials of atrial and ventricular myocardial cells consist of five distinct phases (0 to 4) underlying distinct ionic currents, while there are only three phases in pacemaker cells (0,3,4) (Figures 4a, b):

- phase 0 (upstroke and rapid depolarization) determined by rapid inflow sodium current (I_{Na+});
- phase 1 (early rapid depolarization) caused by inactivation of the sodium current and activation of the outward K$^+$ current (I_{to} K$^+$) and inward initial Ca^{++} current (I_{Ca++}) through transient and long-lasting voltage-dependent channels (T- and L-type);
- phase 2 (plateau) due to persistent inward Ca^{++} currents (L-type channel), favoring the intracellular Ca^{++} release from sarcoplasmic stores;
- phase 3 (final rapid repolarization), caused by the activation of K$^+$ outward delayed rectifier current (I_K).
- phase 4 (resting membrane potential), which is relatively steady in atrial, ventricular myocardial, and His-Purkinje fibers, but not in pacemaker cells, particularly in the sinoatrial node. The slow diastolic depolarization that confers the typical electrophysiological property of these cells (automatism) is due to several ionic currents which bring the membrane potential from the most hyperpolarized level up to the threshold level that triggers the action potential: decay of outward potassium current (I_K), activation of low-threshold transient type Ca^{++} current (I_{Ca},T) and high-threshold long lasting type Ca^{++} current (I_{Ca},L) and activation of time-dependent mixed Na$^+$-K$^+$ inward current (I_f).

According to different authors, the I_f current, which is activated by hyperpolarization, is one of the most important ionic currents for the regulation of pacemaker cell depolarization (Irisawa et al, 1993; DiFrancesco 1995a). The control of the slope of diastolic depolarization is physiologically influenced by neuroautonomic activity which acts particularly on the I_f current, which is inhibited or excited by cholinergic or adrenergic stimulation, respectively (DiFrancesco and Tromba, 1987; DiFrancesco 1995b; Guth and Dietze, 1995).

TRADITIONAL PHARMACOLOGICAL AGENTS

A number of agents have been used in the past in an attempt to control ventricular rate in the failing heart. The most widely used are cardiac glycosides whose beneficial effects in patients with CHF are associated with a reduction in ventricular rate: indeed, acute administration has an immediate sympatho-inhibitory effect and enhances vagal tone; chronic therapy is associated with a sustained decrease in plasma norepinephrine concentrations and increases HRV (Brouwer et al, 1995; Faplan et al, 1997). Amiodarone, an antiarrhythmic agent with minimal negative inotropic effects, also reduces heart rate in patients with atrial fibrillation or in sinus rhythm and increases ejection fraction and exercise tolerance compared with placebo in patients with CHF (Hamer et al, 1989).

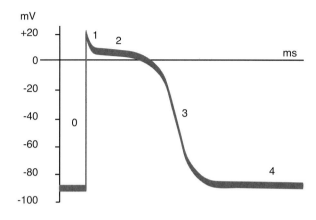

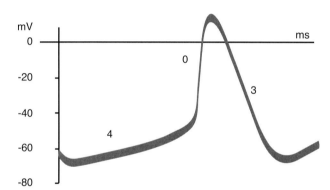

Figure 4. Action potential of common myocardial cells (a) and pacemaker cells (b) (see text for details).

Long-term therapy with β-adrenoceptor blockers also improves hemodynamics and exercise capacity and reduces symptoms of CHF (Jessup, 1991; Lechat et al, 1998; Anderson et al, 1991; Gilbert et al, 1990; Waagstein et al, 1993; CIBIS Investigators, 1994). The beneficial effect of β-blocker therapy is associated with sinus and atrioventricular node cell modulation (through reduction in the rate of phase 4 diastolic depolarization of the action potential) and with prevention of chronic or repetitive ischemia in those patients whose CHF is secondary to coronary artery disease. However, β-blockade also increases HRV, due to its known capacity to reduce sympathetic nerve activity. Furthermore, these agents also reduce arrhythmias (Heilbrunn et al, 1989; Gilbert et al, 1990). Indirect evidence that the damping effects of adrenergic stimulation by β-blockers is beneficial comes from the use of catecholamines (ibopamine, dobutamine) and phosphodiesterase inhibitors (amrinone, milrinone) in patients with CHF. These agents, by increasing heart rate and facilitating arrhythmias, exert potentially harmful effects during long-term therapy and worsen prognosis (Packer et al, 1991).

However, β-blockers are a heterogeneous class of agents. First-generation molecules (such as propranolol) are not selective and, despite reducing heart rate, produce a severe decline in cardiac output because they block both β_1- and β_2-receptors and increase systemic vascular resistance by acting on vascular β_2-receptors.

In contrast, second-generation β_1-selective agents, like metoprolol or bisoprolol, favorably affect both hemodynamics and symptoms in patients with CHF. These drugs induce myocardial β-receptor "upregulation" and, by so doing, increase myocyte sensitivity to the adrenergic drive. Moreover, they have no effect on the β_2-peripheral vascular receptors whose vasodilatator activity counteracts their negative inotropic effects.

Third-generation agents (e.g., carvedilol) have been shown to yield a greater protection because they block β_1- and β_2-receptors (but do not upregulate β_1-receptors) and also possess vasodilatator activity which is due to α_1-adrenoreceptor blockade in the case of carvedilol.

Several items of data suggest that potential differences exist between second- and third-generation agents in patients with CHF: the greater effect of carvedilol is perhaps correlated with the inadequate doses that were used in the earlier trials employing second-generation agents (Heidenreich et al, 1997; CIBIS II Investigators, 1999; MERIT-HF Study Group, 1999). An ongoing multicenter trial is evaluating this hypothesis.

Calcium-channel blockers (diltiazem, verapamil, and gallopamil) also modulate heart rate favorably by acting on the long-lasting, voltage-dependent Ca^{++} channel, thereby inhibiting the influx Ca^{++} current during phases 1 and 2 of the action potential in myocardial fibers and during diastolic phase 4 in pacemaker cells, thus reducing their firing rate. Nevertheless, the suppression of the Ca^{++} current reduces the sarcoplasmic Ca^{++} concentration and impairs myocardial contractility. Initial clinical observations made in severe CHF demonstrated that intravenous and short-term oral diltiazem improves left ventricular performance and reduces myocardial oxygen demand by decreasing heart rate and afterload. However, although no immediate effects on contractile function were observed in this study (Walsh et al, 1984), the chronic use of non-dihydropyridine Ca^{++} blockers in patients with CHF is not recommended in patients with CHF because of their potential long-term negative inotropic effects.

SINUS NODE MODULATORS

Recently, pharmacological modulation of heart rate using new agents without negative inotropic properties has been proposed. Among the different agents, the potassium-channel blocker tedisamil has been investigated extensively but has not been introduced into clinical practice because it causes a number of untoward effects involving the peripheral as well as the pulmonary circulation. Of the other specific bradycardic compounds, the so-called "sinus node modulators", zatebradine, the prototypical molecule, has not fulfilled safety criteria and has been withdrawn; the novel compound ivabradine is undergoing phase 3 clinical evaluation and appears a promising heart rate–lowering drug.

Tedisamil, the first direct bradycardic agent ever tested in humans, exerts anti-ischemic and anti-arrhythmic effects by blocking the repolarization K^+ outward currents during phase 1 (I_{to}) and 3 (I_K) of the action potential. The drug induces a dose-dependent decrease in heart rate by acting directly on the sinus node, thereby reducing myocardial oxygen consumption. It causes a dose-dependent prolongation of cardiac repolarization through an increase in both the relative and effective refractory period which lengthens the QTc interval on the surface ECG. As a result, tedisamil, like amiodarone, is considered to belong to the Class III antiarrhythmic agents.

The compound was hypothesized to be useful in heart failure because of its potent bradycardic action and the lack of significant inotropic effects. However, Hermann et al (1998) observed that intravenous administration of tedisamil, besides causing a significant reduction in heart rate, also increased mean blood pressure and systemic vascular resistance as well as pulmonary artery and capillary wedge pressures and vascular resistance. The mechanism responsible for these effects is probably related to its specific mode of action. In fact, suppression of outward-directed K^+ I_{to} and I_K currents is associated with increased calcium influx in vasculature smooth muscle cells due to inhibition of distinct calcium-sensitive and ATP-sensitive potassium channels (I_{KATP}).

In the early nineties, drugs with a new pharmacological profile were described as "specific bradycardic agents." They decrease heart rate by direct interaction with the pacemaker cells of the sinoatrial node. Electrophysiologically they induce a reduction in the rate of diastolic depolarization of phase 4 of the action potential by blocking the hyperpolarization-activated I_f current, without affecting maximal diastolic or threshold potential.

Among these drugs, zatebradine (UL-FS 469), a molecule chemically related to verapamil, was the first one to be studied (Goethals et al, 1993). The agent is a nonselective I_f current inhibitor in the sinoatrial node, that also blocks the $Ca^{++}{}_{T,L}$ and rectifies outward K^+ currents (Bois et al, 1996). As a result, zatebradine prolongs action potential duration in pig papillary muscle and in rabbit Purkinje fibers (Valenzuela et al, 1996). In the intact anesthetized pig, zatebradine also inhibits, in a dose-dependent way, the increase in heart rate induced by administration of isoproterenol or norepinephrine, without affecting β-receptor–mediated increases in myocardial contractility (Guth and Dietze, 1995). In the conscious rabbit, where heart failure had been induced by rapid atrial pacing, zatebradine decreased heart rate without affecting left ventricular function (Ryu et al, 1996). However, in human subjects, apart from reducing sinus rate, acute intravenous administration of zatebradine prolongs the conduction and refractory properties of the atrioventricular node, but has no effect on atrial refractoriness, His-Purkinje conduction, ventricular refractoriness, and action potential duration (Chiamvimonat et al, 1998). In patients with moderate left ventricular dysfunction, oral zatebradine did not decrease contractility, increased cardiac external work without increasing myocardial oxygen consumption, and resulted in improved mechanical efficiency (Shinke et al, 1999).

Unfortunately, the clinical use of this interesting agent was hampered by an exceedingly high incidence of adverse visual phenomena both in patients and volunteers. As a result, zatebradine was withdrawn and never reached the pharmaceutical market.

Recently, a novel heart rate-reducing agent, ivabradine, has been described (Thollon et al, 1994). In rabbit sinoatrial node preparations, ivabradine reduces the spontaneous action potential firing rate of pacemaker cells by reducing the diastolic depolarization slope and prolonging the diastolic depolarization time (see Figure 5a).

Ivabradine selectively inhibits the pacemaker I_f current in a dose-dependent way and has no effect on either $I_{Ca^{++}T}$, nor $I_{Ca^{++}L}$ currents. Therefore, the heart rate-reducing effect is not mediated by inhibition of Ca^{++} currents (especially of the L-type), which explains the absence of the negative inotropic effect, typical of these drugs (Goethals et al, 1993).

Ivabradine has negligible effects on action potential duration (phase 3) in therapeutically relevant doses both in sinoatrial and ventricular cells (see Figures 5b-c) (Thollon et al, 1997). This represents a major advantage as the prolongation of action potential, especially if associated with a low heart rate, may favor the occurrence of early afterdepolarizations, triggering malignant polymorphic ventricular tachyarrhythmias. Thus, ivabradine, an agent devoid of direct effect on action potential repolarization, is likely to be safer in clinical use.

Furthermore, ivabradine decreases heart rate and markedly increases HRV in conscious rats. However, when given after sympathovagal blockade, obtained with atropine plus propranolol, the drug still causes bradycardia accompanied with a reduction in HRV. This observation confirms that the inverse correlation between heart rate and HRV is not an intrinsic property of pacemaker cells but is dependent on the balance between the two components of the neuroautonomic system (Mangin et al, 1998). Therefore, the increase in HRV that is observed when ivabradine is given alone, reflects the reduction in sympathetic activity indirectly caused by the improvement in cardiocirculatory function produced by the drug.

Ivabradine does not significantly influence hemodynamic parameters such as myocardial contractility or blood pressure (Simon et al, 1995). Furthermore, ivabradine improves the recovery of contractility in a dog model of left ventricular dysfunction induced by ischemia (Monnet et al, 2001). The heart rate-reducing dose-dependent properties of the agent have also been confirmed in healthy volunteers: the N-dealkylated metabolite contributes to this effect (Ragueneau et al, 1998).

CONCLUSIONS

Reducing heart rate is a critical target to achieve in the presence of myocardial dysfunction, in order to maintain sufficient systolic tension which, in failing hearts, is further reduced by the "inverse" force-frequency relationship.

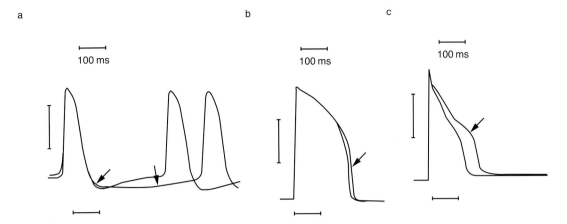

FIGURE 5. Effect of ivabradine (stereoisomer S16257) on phase 4 of rabbit sinoatrial preparation action potential (a), on phase 3 of guinea-pig papillary muscles (b) and rabbit Purkinje fiber (c) (see arrows). Modified with permission from Thollon et al, 1997.

Excessive tachycardia that is generally seen in patients with severe heart failure is a marker of depressed left ventricular function and reflects abnormal activation of the sympathetic nervous system. Thus, heart rate modulation would appear useful for reducing myocardial oxygen consumption and prolonging diastolic filling and coronary perfusion time.

The beneficial effects of long-term β-blocker treatment in dilated cardiomyopathy are thought to be related to both reduction in heart rate and to partial inhibition of the neurohormonal cascade that is caused by sympathetic stimulation and favors the progression of left ventricular failure through a number of cardiac and systemic effects. However, the use of full therapeutic doses of β-blockers is often limited in clinical practice by the concomitant decrease in contractile function caused by ventricular $β_1$-receptor blockade.

Sinoatrial rate modulators are potent heart rate–reducing drugs acting by inhibition of the pacemaker I_f current. Since the latter plays a key role under conditions of increased adrenergic tone, these compounds and particularly ivabradine, a highly specific agent that inhibits this current and lacks negative inotropic effects, may represent a valuable pharmacological tool for the treatment of left ventricular systolic dysfunction expecially when caused by chronic myocardial ischemia.

CHAPTER 12

HEART RATE REDUCTION AND MORBIDITY AND MORTALITY IN CARDIOVASCULAR DISORDERS

BRAMAH N. SINGH

INTRODUCTION

Over the last two decades or so, an increasing number of prospective and retrospective primary and secondary observational studies have analyzed the nature of the association between heart rate and coronary artery disease, myocardial infarction, and hypertension (Dyer et al, 1980; Hinkle, 1981; Kannel et al; 1985,1987; Gillum, 1988; Gillum et al, 1991; Hjalmarson et al, 1990; Hjalmarson, 1990; Gillman et al, 1993; Kjekshus, 1985, 1986; Singh, 1999). In these clinical settings as in others, sustained elevated heart rate has emerged as a highly predictive factor for a significantly higher rate of total mortality (Kjekshus, 1985; Hjalmarson et al, 1990; Hjalmarson, 1990) compared with subjects in whom the heart rate is persistently in the normal or a lower range.

Over the same period, consistently favorable effects of β-blockade on mortality and morbidity have been confirmed in large blinded placebo-controlled clinical trials in post–myocardial infarction patients as well as in those with congestive heart failure (CIBIS II Investigators and Committees, 1999; MERIT-HF Study Group, 1999; Packer, 1998; Packer et al, 2001). Such beneficial effects have been noted to correlate significantly with their heart rate–lowering actions (Kjekshus, 1985, 1986) providing a compelling rationale for exploring the potential therapeutic role of other heart rate–lowering agents in cardiovascular disorders. In this regard, the pharmacologic action of the blockers of the sinus pacemaker current (I_f), the so-called specific heart rate–lowering agents (DiFrancesco, 1993), may be of particular importance as anti-ischemic agents while having the potential for reducing morbidity and mortality in cardiovascular disorders especially those characterized by sustained and significant elevations in heart rate (Singh and Vanhoutte, 2002). In this chapter, the clinical settings in which increased heart rate may be an independent risk factor for cardiovascular morbidity and mortality will be critically discussed and placed in perspective for the evolution of pharmacologic therapy to attenuate the observed risk.

SUSTAINED INCREASES IN HEART RATE AS A PREDICTOR OF RISK FOR CARDIOVASCULAR DISORDERS: EPIDEMIOLOGICAL OBSERVATIONS

A number of epidemiological studies have examined the relationship between resting heart rate and mortality in patients with coronary artery disease, myocardial infarction, and hypertension as well as in patients without evidence of cardiovascular disease and attendant mortality. The outcome data are directionally consistent. The bulk of the analysis has been derived from the databases of the Framingham Heart Study (Kannel et al, 1985, 1987), the first National Health and Nutrition Examination Survey or NHANES I (Gillum, 1988), in particular the NHANES I Epidemiological Follow-up Study or NNHEFS (Gillum et al, 1991), the Chicago Employee Studies (Dyer et al, 1980), the Goteborg Primary Prevention Trial (Wilhelmsen et al, 1986), and the CORDIS study (Green and Peled, 1992; Kristal-Boneh et al, 2000). Only those aspects of the findings in these studies that deal with the seemingly direct impact of increased heart rate relative to mortality and morbidity will be discussed. Disease-specific effects relative to hypertension and post–myocardial infarction patients are discussed in a later section of this chapter.

HEART RATE AND CARDIOVASCULAR MORTALITY

The longest follow-up has been reported from the Framingham Heart Study, a prospective study which was started in 1948 (Kannel et al, 1987). The report on the relationship between heart rate and

TABLE 1. Overall deaths by resting heart rates relative to age and gender: 30-year follow-up Framingham study

	AGE-ADJUSTED ANNUAL INCIDENCE/1000			
	MEN (YEARS)		WOMEN (YEARS)	
RESTING HEART RATE (BPM)	35–64**	65–94**	35–64***	65–94*
30–67	6	35	3	22
68–75	8	43	4	28
76–83	11	46	6	25
84–91	13	61	8	30
92–220	24	64	9	35

Trends for significance: $*P < 0.05$; $**P < 0.01$; $***P < 0.001$. Adapted from Kannel et al, 1987

TABLE 2. Sudden death by heart rate according to age in men: 30-year follow-up in Framingham Study

	AGE-ADJUSTED ANNUAL INCIDENCE/1000			
	PERSONS FREE OF PRIOR CORONARY ARTERY DISEASE (YEARS)		ALL PERSONS ALIVE (YEARS)	
RESTING HEART RATE (BPM)	35–64**	65–94**	35–64***	65–94*
30–67	1	2	1	4
68–75	1	3	1	4
76–83	1	4	2	7
84–91	2	7	3	12
92–220	3	6	5	6

Trends for significance: $*P < 0.05$; $**P < 0.01$; $***P < 0.001$.

cardiovascular mortality focused on 5070 study participants who were free of cardiac disease at entry. They were subjected to a biennial examination of a wide range of variables which included cardiovascular examination and history, an ECG, measurement of vital capacity, body weight, skinfold thickness, various blood chemistry and blood pressure determinations, and elicitation of the history of smoking. The resting ECG was used for the determination of heart rate. Over the follow-up period of 30 years, there were 1876 total deaths; of these, 894 deaths were cardiovascular in origin. For both sexes, all-cause, cardiovascular, and coronary disease mortality increased progressively as a function of the antecedent resting heart rates determined biennially. There was no suggestion of critical values or threshold of heart rates which could be labeled as safe or hazardous. The trend significance was at $P < 0.01$ as it was for sudden death as presented in Tables 1 and 2 and in Figure 1. The effects of heart rate both on total mortality as well as on sudden death were independent of associated cardiovascular risk factors and the correlation between higher death rate and elevated heart rate was higher in males than in females.

Kannel and his colleagues (1987) noted that the case fatality rates following coronary events were also higher in patients with augmented heart rates. Of particular interest, there was a large excess of noncardiovascular deaths at high heart rates which, as the authors suggested, lends credence to the notion that heart rate may be a nonspecific measure of health and mortality rates, a concept that has therapeutic implications. In this context, another feature from the Framingham study should be emphasized. Goldberg et al (1996) followed 747 men and 973 women beyond the age of 50 years, after those who had diabetes, cardiovascular disease, and cancer had been excluded. They used a logistic regression

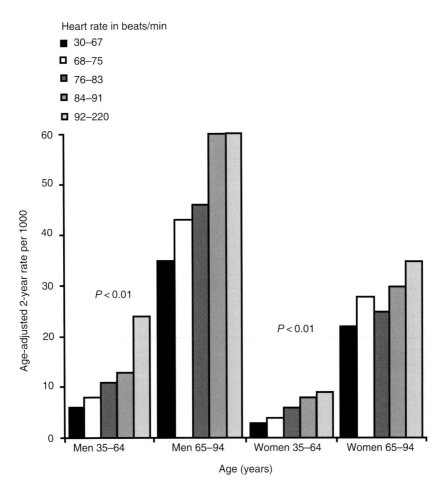

Figure 1 Overall deaths relative to heart rate according to age and gender: Follow-up Framingham Study. Note that the age-adjusted 2-year rate per 1000 study participants shows a significant trend in mortality as the heart rate increases. The death rate is higher in males than in females at every decile of observation. See text for details. Adapted from Kannel et al, 1987.

statistical model to examine factors associated with survival to 75 years of age. Among other factors such as lighter cigarette smoking, lower blood pressure, and higher forced vital capacity, they found lower heart rate in men and parental survival to 75 years of age in women were additionally associated with survival to 75 years of age.

The relationship between heart rate, coronary artery disease, and death was also investigated systematically in the NHANES I Epidemiologic Follow-up Study or NHEFS (Gillum, 1988; Gillum et al, 1991). The participants in this study were screened from those who were 25–74 years of age at the time of the initial survey in 1971–1975. From the initial 7594 patients at baseline, 5136 white and 859 black patients (aged between 45 and 74 years) remained for analysis after all defined exclusion criteria were met and follow-up variables established. The duration of follow-up for this analysis was from 6–13 years, average 9.9 years for white patients and 10.3 years for the black survivors.

It is noteworthy that, in contrast to the Framingham Study, heart rates were not quantified by an ECG but were obtained by a physician who counted the radial pulse for 30 s. The relative risk (RR) for the incidence of coronary heart disease (CHD) was elevated significantly in white men with the pulse rate >84 beats/min compared with those with rates <74 beats/min after correcting for multiple risk factors. The incidence of CHD was also increased in white women with elevated pulse rate. The risks for death from all causes, cardiovascular diseases, and noncardiovascular diseases were also elevated for white men with raised pulse rate independent of other factors. It should be emphasized that the risks of death and cardiovascular diseases were also increased in the case of black men and women with elevated pulse rate. However, the association of cardiovascular disease with high pulse rate was particularly striking in the case of black women even after the adjustment for all the baseline risk factors.

Similar data on the incidence of all-cause mortality as well as CHD mortality, and total mortality, have been found in the Goteborg Primary Prevention Trial in Sweden (Wilhelmsen et al, 1986). This study was a prospective one in which the effects of a multifactorial intervention program on CHD, stroke incidence, and total mortality as well as cardiovascular mortality were determined. The intervention group included 10 000 men and the two control groups were of a similar number.

The intervention included dietary measures for elevated serum cholesterol, blood pressure treatment if screen levels demonstrated significantly high levels, and advice for the smokers in the study population. The intervention was applied for over 10 years. The data suggested a benefit in terms of reduction in total mortality, stroke, and CHD for not only the intervention group but also the two control groups, indicating overall reduction in the major risk factors in the general male population of Goteborg in Sweden. However, of the 7455 study patients in whom the heart rate data were available in the registry and followed for a mean of 11.8 years, deaths were stratified into total mortality, death due to coronary artery disease, cancer, stroke, and other deaths and correlated with the initial heart rates. The follow-up data are presented in Figure 2. It is noteworthy that the rate of death from all causes and from cardiovascular disease increased as a function of increasing heart rate or when pulse rate was ≥84 beats/min as has been reported in the NHANES I Epidemiologic Follow-up Study (Gillum, 1988).

IMPACT OF HEART RATE VARIATIONS IN STUDIES IN INDUSTRY EMPLOYEES

Two studies confined to industry employees have been reported. In the first of these, the Chicago Cohort Study (Dyer et al, 1980), heart rate as a prognostic factor for CHD and for mortality was determined in three distinct epidemiological studies 20 years ago. The associations between heart rate and death from cardiovascular diseases, coronary artery disease, sudden cardiac death from CHD as well as mortality from all causes were studied prospectively in middle-aged white male employees. The patient distribution in each of the three studies was as follows: (a) 1899 men aged 40–55 years from Chicago Western Electric Company followed for 17 years, (b) 1233 men aged 40–59 years from Chicago Peoples Gas Company followed for 15 years, and (c) 5784 men aged 45–64 years of age from the Chicago Heart Association Detection Project in Industry followed for five years. In a univariate analysis, mortality from cardiovascular or noncardiovascular causes rose with increasing heart rate in all three studies. In a multivariate Cox regression analysis, controlling for hypertension, age, serum cholesterol, number of cigarettes smoked per day, and relative weight, heart rate emerged as a significant risk factor for sudden death in two of the three studies.

In sum, the authors concluded that the results of the three studies suggested that high heart rate may be an independent risk factor for sudden death from CHD. A similar study has been reported by Kristal-Boneh et al (2000) in Israeli industrial employees. They reported the data relating resting heart rate at entry as a predictor of coronary artery disease mortality in an 8-year follow-up evaluation of 3527 male study participants who were under observation in the so-called Cardiovascular Occupational Risk Factor Determination in Israel (CORDIS) study (Green and Peled, 1992). During follow-up, there were 135 deaths, 57 from cardiovascular disease and 45 from cancer, the remaining deaths being of miscellaneous origins. They found that heart rates ≥90 beats/min at entry into the study had an adjusted relative risk of 2.23 (95% CI, 1.4–3.6) compared with those whose heart rates were <70 beats/min (Green and Peled, 1992) after the data had been adjusted in various statistical models allowing for various risk factors and biochemical parameters. A similar result was found in the case of cardiovascular mortality with a relative risk of 2.02 (95% CI, 1.1–4.0) but there was no effect on cancer mortality as has been reported in a different study by Wilhelmsen et al (1986).

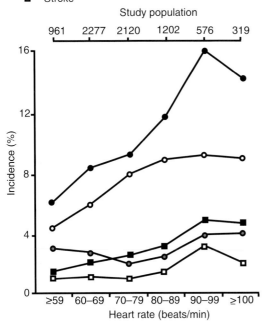

Figure 2 The incidence of mortality from various causes over a mean period of 11.8 years of follow-up as a function of heart rate at entry to the Goteborg Primary Prevention Trial. The study population refers to the number of patients within a range of heart rates at entry. Note that there is a steep increase in total as well as coronary heart disease mortality as a function of heart rate increase but this did not occur in the case of cancer. See text for details. Adapted from Wilhelmsen et al, 1986.

HEART RATE AND MORTALITY PATTERNS IN HYPERTENSION AND POST–MYOCARDIAL INFARCTION

The data relating the effects of variations in heart rate on total mortality as well as cardiovascular mortality are perhaps of the greatest importance clinically in the setting of hypertension and in patients with known coronary artery disease syndromes, especially those sustaining and surviving myocardial infarction. In the USA alone, there are 50–60 million hypertensive individuals and about 1.5 million of these develop acute myocardial infarction.

RISK OF HIGH HEART RATE IN HYPERTENSION AND IN THE ELDERLY

It is known that hypertensive patients generally have a higher heart rate than comparable normotensive patients (Gillum,1988). Gillman et al (1993) followed 4530 hypertensive patients, aged between 35 and 74 years with BP ≥140 mmHg systolic and ≥90 mmHg diastolic, for 36 years from the Framingham Heart Study. During the follow-up period, in individuals who had increases in heart rates exceeding 40 beats/min, the total mortality more than doubled over this period. The details are summarized in Figure 3. The rapid heart rate that the patients had was not related to pre-existing illness but appeared to be an independent risk factor for cardiovascular death in patients with hypertension. Thus, the heart rate data relative to the impact on mortality are consistent with those reported for patients with known CHD (Kannel et al, 1987; Gillum et al, 1991) and those for patients who had sustained but survived myocardial infarction as discussed below (Hjalmarson et al,1990). The data suggest that the treatment regimens for hypertension may need to include heart rate-lowering drugs. Also of interest are the outcomes of the study reported by Aronow et al (1996). They evaluated the risk of high heart rate in the elderly patients (60–100 years; mean age, 81 years) who had hypertensive or other forms of heart disease but were in

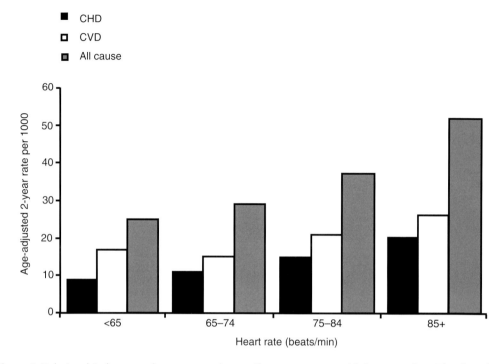

Figure 3 Relationship between heart rate and mortality among men with hypertension. The data that form the basis of this bar diagram were derived from a 36-year follow-up of the Framingham Heart Study. CHD=coronary heart disease; CVD=cardiovascular heart disease. See text for details. Based on the data from Gillman et al, 1993.

normal sinus rhythm. It was a prospective study in which 1311 patients whose mean heart rates were quantified from 24-h Holter recordings. The authors found that male gender, increasing age, and the mean 24-h heart rates were independent risk factors for new coronary events. The probability of developing new coronary events was 1.14 times higher for an increment of 5 beats/min of heart rate after the effects of other confounding risk factors were controlled for.

Myocardial infarction, high heart rate, and mortality

There have been a number of studies that have documented two features of clinical importance: (i) the overall heart rate in patients sustaining myocardial infarction is higher (mean 78.5 beats/min) than that (69.5 beats/min) in matched controls, and (ii) elevated heart rate in individuals is predictive of the risk for their developing acute myocardial infarction (AMI) and sustaining complications while having a greater risk of death (Hjalmarson et al, 1990). Furthermore, the sustained elevated heart rate in patients after AMI correlates well with higher mortality (Gundersen et al, 1986). The results of a relatively large study involving 1807 post–myocardial infarction patients reported by Hjalmarson (1990) are the most germane to the current discussion. In a multicenter study, they examined heart rate on admission to the coronary care unit and at discharge and correlated the heart rates with the total mortality from day two to one year in patients with and without heart failure. The mortality figures from hospital discharge to one year at increasing maximal heart rate values and values observed at discharge physical examination are presented in Figure 4. In patients with severe grades of heart failure, the cumulative mortality was high (61–68%) regardless of the level of admission heart rate. Thus, the question arises as to whether the high mortality rates associated with increases in heart rates can be attenuated by heart rate reduction.

TABLE 3. Results of some end-point trials of β-blockers in patients after myocardial infarction and in heart failure

TRIAL/DRUG	N	β-BLOCKER	TOTAL MORTALITY REDUCTION	SUDDEN DEATH REDUCTION
CUMULATIVE (post MI)	>50 000	Various	23% ($P < 0.01$)	23% ($P < 0.001$)
BHAT-CHF	710	Propranolol	27% ($P < 0.05$)	28% ($P < 0.05$)
MC Carvedilol trials	1094	Carvedilol	65% ($P < 0.001$)	55% ($P < 0.001$)
CIBIS-II	2647	Bisoprolol	34% ($P < 0.001$)	44% ($P = 0.0011$)
MERIT-HF	3991	Metoprolol	34% ($P = 0.0002$)	34% ($P = 0.0002$)
COPERNICUS	2289	Carvedilol	35% ($P = 0.0014$)	41% ($P = 0.0001$)
BEST	2708	Bucindolol	8% (NS)	10% (NS)

Post MI, Post myocardial infarction; NS, not significant; NR, not reported. Adapted from Reiter, 2000.

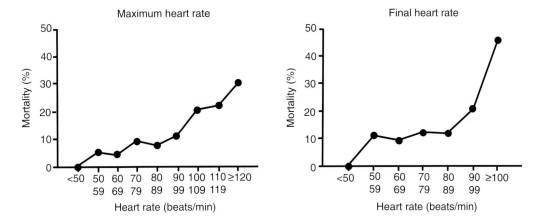

Figure 4 Mortality from discharge to one year at maximal heart rate values observed at discharge physical examination. The data are from a follow-up of 1807 postinfarction patients with heart rates obtained at the time of admission for the acute event, and at the time of hospital discharge. The follow-up data were obtained from day two of the infarction and to 12 months thereafter. Note that heart rate of 80 beats/min appears to be the threshold for increase in mortality. Adapted from Hjalmarson et al (1990).

LESSONS FROM β-BLOCKER TRIALS

As a class of drugs, β-blockers produce a distinctive effect in consistently reducing heart rate by blocking β-adrenergic receptors in the sinus node. The precise magnitude of such an effect varies with the dose of an individual drug as well as with the degree of intrinsic sympathomimetic effects the compound concurrently might have. Whether this is a cause-and-effect relationship is unclear but heart rate reduction is associated with beneficial therapeutic effects in acute as well as chronic myocardial ischemic syndromes and, importantly, prolongation of survival in a wide variety of cardiovascular disorders including heart failure. These observations are in line with those indicating that β-blockade has the proclivity to prevent the development of ventricular fibrillation in a variety of experimental animal models (Singh, 1990; Meredith et al, 1991; Reiter and Reiffel, 1998; Reiter, 2000). However, in the clinic, the antiarrhythmic potential of β-blockade was greatly overshadowed by its anti-ischemic actions for which this class of drugs was synthesized in the 1960s. On the other hand, that the increased activity of the sympathetic nervous system with marked elevations in heart rate might induce cardiovascular morbidity and mortality through a variety of mechanisms has been known for many years (Reiter, 2000; Kjekshus, 1985,

1986). For example, given the appropriate pathologic substrate, increased sympathetic activity may be associated with sudden arrhythmic death (Eliot and Buell, 1985; Julius, 1993; Leenen, 1999). This is now known to be particularly striking in the case of patients developing myocardial infarction with or without heart failure (Yusuf et al, 1985; Singh, 1990; Packer, 1998).

The electrophysiologic consequences of sympathetic hyperactivity have been extensively documented in numerous experimental and clinical studies (Kannel et al, 1985; Julius, 1993; Singh, 1998, 1999). In the experimental arena they have included, (i) shortening of the ventricular action potential duration, and hence the refractory period, (ii) augmenting ventricular conduction, (iii) increasing ventricular automaticity, (iv) reducing vagal tone (James et al, 1977), (v) decreasing ventricular fibrillation threshold, and (vi) reversing or attenuating the effects of antiarrhythmic drugs administered in the expectation of preventing arrhythmic deaths. Conversely, it is known that the depletion of the adrenergic transmitters to the heart increases ventricular fibrillation (VF) threshold and in experimental models in which VF could be induced reproducibly, the arrhythmia is preventable by sympathetic blockade (Singh 1990; Leenen, 1999; Singh, 1999). It is known that, as a class, β-adrenergic blocking drugs are effective in reducing mortality in many subsets of patients with manifest arrhythmias and in those at high risk for dying from arrhythmic deaths (Schwartz, 1985; Tan et al, 1995; Wiesfeld et al, 1996; Steinbeck et al, 1992; Hallstrom et al, 1991; Kendall et al, 1995; Hjalmarson, 1997). The impact has been sudden death in patients with congenital long QT interval syndrome, in survivors of cardiac arrest, and in selected cases of ventricular tachycardia. However, the outcome data from the double-blinded, placebo-controlled trials in patients after myocardial infarction and those with congestive heart failure are the most compelling. There have been no antiarrhythmic agents which have been shown to produce such a consistent and significant reduction in mortality as have β-blockers in the survivors of myocardial infarction nor in those with congestive heart failure. A number of therapeutic implications that stem from these findings may have significant clinical implications. In the case of the post–myocardial infarction patients, total mortality as well as arrhythmia mortality as judged by the reduced incidence of sudden death were found to be significantly lowered (Kendall et al, 1995; Hjalmarson, 1997). They also produced a consistent and significant reduction in the incidence of myocardial reinfarction (Habib, 1997; Hallstrom et al, 1991).

Recent trials have focused on congestive heart failure (Packer, 1998; Bristow, 2000). There have been three decisive trials which have confirmed a highly significant effect on total mortality and on sudden death. The salient parameters are presented in Table 3 in which the data on the post-MI patients are also included. In the trial involving the use of metoprolol in 3991 patients with largely class II–IV New York Heart Association (NYHA) heart failure (left ventricular ejection fraction<40%), randomized to long-acting metoprolol ($n = 1990$) in graduated doses up to 200 mg/day or placebo ($n = 2001$), the primary end point was all-cause mortality, analyzed by intention to treat. The mean follow-up was one year. During the period of follow-up, there were 147 deaths (7.2%) on metoprolol versus 217 deaths (11.0%) on placebo. This difference was significant ($P < 0.00009$). There was a statistically significant reduction in sudden death on metoprolol when compared with that on placebo (MERIT-HF Study Group, 1999).

Similar data have been reported for the drug bisoprolol in 2647 patients in a double-blind, multi-center study (CIBIS II Investigators and Committees, 1999) with randomization to the β-blocker ($n = 1327$) or placebo ($n = 1320$). The patients, all in class III–IV CHF with a left ventricular ejection fraction of 35% or lower, were taking diuretics and angiotensin-converting enzyme (ACE) inhibitors as in the case of the MERIT-HF trial. All-cause mortality was 11.8% (156 deaths) versus 17.3% (17.3%). This difference was significant ($P < 0.0001$). The drug was effective in reducing sudden death significantly. The third trial involves the use of carvedilol (Packer et al, 2001) in which 2289 largely class II to class IV patients were randomized to placebo or carvedilol with a target drug dose of 2 mg bid, and a starting dose of 6.125 mg bid. The mean left ventricular ejection fraction of the total number of patients enrolled in the study was 19.8%. At the end of the study, the placebo mortality was 18.5%, and the mortality on carvedilol 11.4%, a risk reduction of 35% ($P = 0.00013$). The sudden death rate reduction was about 40%. Thus, it is clear that in patients after myocardial infarction as well as in patients with significant heart failure, β-blockade reduces cardiovascular as well as total mortality in addition to sudden cardiac death.

TABLE 4. Clinical consequences of high heart rate and implications of reducing heart rate for clinical outcome

HEART RATE	IMPACT	POPULATION
>84 beats/min at rest	Elevated risk of CHD	White men aged 65 to 74 years White women aged 45 to 74 years (Gillman et al, 1993)
Increase ≥40 beats/min	>twofold higher all-cause mortality	Hypertensive subjects (Gillman et al, 1993)
50-69 beats/min on admission	15% total mortality at 1 year post-MI	AMI patients (Hjalmarson et al, 1990)
≥90 beats/min on admission	30% total mortality at 1 year post-MI	AMI patients (as above)
>110 beats/min on admission	48% total mortality at 1 year post-MI	AMI patients (as above)
<90 beats/min	5-7% severe heart failure	AMI patients (as above)
≥90 beats/min on admission	24% severe heart failure	AMI patients (as above)
14-beat/min decrement with β-blocker therapy within 12 h of symptom onset	25-30% decreased infarct size	AMI patients (Kjekshus, 1986)
5-beat/min increment in heart rate	1.14 higher probability coronary events	Men and women; mean age 81 years (Aronow, 1996)
>90 bpm compared to <70 bpm	2.23 increase in relative risk for death	Industrial employees, in CORDIS study

CHD, coronary heart disease; MI, myocardial infarction; AMI, acute myocardial infarction. Adapted from Habib, 1997.

As far as the β-blocker trials are concerned, whether they have been in infarct survivors or in congestive cardiac failure, the magnitude of effect on mortality correlates closely to the degree of reduction in heart rate. These correlative data was initially presented by Kjekshus (1985, 1986) in the survivors of myocardial infarction. He pointed out that β-blockers which exerted significant sympathomimetic properties (e.g., oxprenolol, practolol, pindolol) produced proportionately lower degrees of mortality reduction compared with those agents such as metoprolol (MERIT-HF Study Group, 1999), propranolol (β-Blocker Heart Attack Trial Research Group, 1984), and timolol (Norwegian Multicenter Study Group, 1981; Gundersen et al, 1986); acebutolol, which has minimal agonist actions, had an intermediate effect. Of particular interest, sotalol, which produced a marked reduction in heart rate, exerted a modest effect on mortality that did not reach statistical significance (Julian et al, 1982). The reason for this is not entirely clear, but the survival curve in the sotalol study indicated an early increase in mortality compared with placebo. This may have been due to the dosing of the drug as a single-dose regimen of 360 mg daily without adjustment for renal insufficiency or the QT interval. Subsequent heart failure studies with bucindolol (The β-Blocker Evaluation of Survival Trial Investigators, 2001), metoprolol, bisoprolol, and carvedilol (Figure 5) have now confirmed the initial observations made by Kjekshus (1986) linking heart rate reduction and prolongation of survival in patients on β-blocker therapy.

DISCUSSION

Clinical as well as experimental observations reviewed in this chapter provide a convincing basis for the link between elevated heart rate and the development of coronary atherosclerosis (discussed in detail elsewhere in this monograph) with associated increases in all-cause mortality, noncardiovascular mortality as well as cardiovascular mortality. Aspects of the data are summarized in Table 4. Sudden cardiac death and elevated heart rate relationship is perhaps the most compelling (Thaulow and Erikssen, 1991.) Although most studies support the notion that the effect of augmented heart rate is an independent risk factor for cardiovascular mortality and morbidity, this has not been uniform (Dyer et al, 1980; Kannel et al, 1987). For example, heart rate was significantly associated with the incidence of any CHD after adjustment was made for age in men but not for women; in neither was it significant when adjustment was made for

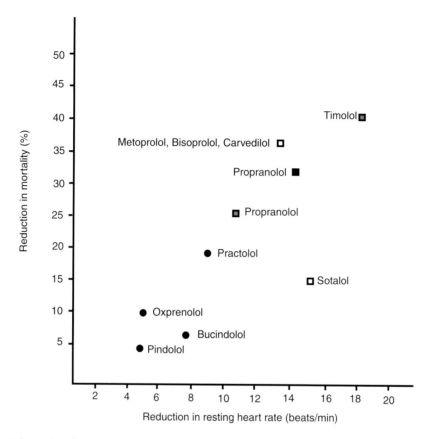

Figure 5 Relationship between reduction in resting heart rate and decrease in mortality in large, prospective, double-blind trials with β-blockers in patients after myocardial infarction and those with congestive heart failure. Circles represent β-blockers with intrinsic sympathomimetic actions. Squares represent β-blockers without intrinsic sympathomimetic actions. Note two studies have been cited for propranolol: the higher value for heart rate reduction and a greater impact in one of these represent the subset of patients with heart failure. It should be noted that metoprolol, bisoprolol, and carvedilol produced an identical percentage reduction in total mortality in patients with congestive heart failure. See text for further details. Adapted from Kjekshus (1985, 1986).

multiple risk factors (Gillum et al, 1991). On the other hand, the association with CHD death and sudden death in men remained significant after adjustment of multiple risk factors (Kannel et al, 1987; Gillum et al, 1991; Stokes et al, 1987). This was also the case in the Chicago cohorts study (Dyer et al, 1980) in regard to sudden CHD death in men aged 45–64 years. The issue in regard to sudden death remained uncertain because of a lack of accurate classification of deaths into sudden versus nonsudden in NHEFS (Gillum et al, 1991) but it was compelling in the case of observations from the Framingham study (Kannel et al, 1987).

There have been some indications regarding gender differences relative to the elevated heart rate as a risk for cardiovascular morbidity and mortality. For example, age-adjusted all-cause mortality and that from cardiovascular diseases were positively correlated with the heart rate in the Chicago Cohort and Framingham Heart studies (Dyer et al, 1980; Kannel et al, 1987). This association was also significant in the case of women in the Framingham Heart Study (Kannel et al, 1987). It is of interest that in both the Framingham as well as Chicago studies there was a positive association between noncardiovascular mortality and elevated heart rate. The findings from the NHEFS (Gillum et al, 1991) are consistent with the data from the studies in which there were associations between CHD and death from all causes and from cardiovascular and noncardiovascular diseases independently of other risk factors. Clearly, further studies are necessary to define more definitively the nature of the relationship between elevated heart rate and the risk for CHD and mortality in women and in African Americans. As suggested by Gillum et al (1991), a clearer delineation is required of the mechanisms of the known associations relative to physical activity, cholesterol status, insulin resistance, left ventricular hypertrophy, as well as continuous measurements of heart rate and blood pressure.

The data summarized in this chapter of the monograph on heart rate and morbidity and mortality may have broader therapeutic implications. It is known that perturbations in heart rate control may occur in a variety of clinical settings in which increases in mortality have been reported. However, a direct link between increases in heart rate in such conditions and associated mortality figures has not been examined critically. For example, sustained elevations of heart rate during casual measurements as well as during the evaluation of its circadian rhythmicity by Holter recordings have indicated higher heart rates in diabetes (Ewing et al, 1981; Ong et al, 1993). This has been attributed to cardiac parasympathetic and sympathetic nervous system damage, a mechanism that may lead to sustained increases in heart rate from an inappropriate autonomic arousal (Eliot and Buell, 1985) and, as has been alluded to, may be associated with sudden cardiac death (Ong et al, 1993). It is also known that in hypertensive patients (Conway, 1984) there often is an increased heart rate as in the case of smokers in whom high heart rate may accelerate the development of atherosclerosis (Aronow, 1978). It has been reported that when patients with angina stop smoking, there is a decrease in heart rate accompanied by a reduction in the extent of ST-T wave changes induced by exercise (McHenry et al, 1977). In the Framingham study, Kannel et al (1987) have shown that the association of rapid heart rate with death persists, taking cigarette smoking and blood pressure into account. Whether a reduction in heart rate by protracted exercise or by β-blockade may improve cardiovascular mortality in general or sudden death in particular in this setting remains to be determined.

Conclusions

In sum, there is now a substantive body of evidence that sustained elevated heart rate is associated with an increased incidence of mortality in patients with suspected or known coronary artery disease, in those with documented myocardial infarction, patients with hypertension, and those who are elderly and have hypertension. Increases in sudden cardiac death have been consistent findings in patients with elevated heart rate. Prophylactic β-blockers at doses at which they significantly reduce heart rate attenuate the attendant risk while reducing the severity of myocardial ischemia in subsets of patients in whom they have been tested. Specific heart rate–lowering agents, as discussed in this monograph, have been developed as antianginal compounds on the basis of their major effects in reducing myocardial oxygen consumption. Moreover, they may have broader clinical therapeutic applications, which merit serious scrutiny in relevant clinical trials. The possibility that the heart rate lowering per se might be the most significant mechanism for reducing mortality, and especially sudden cardiac death, may be resolved by the use of selective I_f inhibitors (DiFrancesco, 1993; Lillie and Singh, 1994) bereft of the property of adrenergic blockade.

REFERENCES

Abi-Gerges N, Ji GJ, Lu ZJ, Fischmeister R, Hescheler J, Fleischmann BK (2000) Functional expression and regulation of the hyperpolarization-activated non-selective cation current in embryonic stem cell-derived cardiomyocytes. *J Physiol.* **523**:377–389.

Abildskov JA (1976) Effects of activation sequence on the local recovery of ventricular excitability in the dog. *Circ Res.* **38**:240–243.

Accili EA, Redaelli G, DiFrancesco D (1996) Activation of the hyperpolarization-activated current (I_f) in sino-atrial node myocytes of the rabbit by vasoactive intestinal peptide. *Pflügers Arch-Eur J Physiol.* **431**:803–805.

Accili EA, Redaelli G, DiFrancesco D (1998) Two distinct pathways of muscarinic current responses in rabbit sino-atrial node myocytes. *Pflügers Arch-Eur J Physiol.* **437**:164–167.

Accili EA, Robinson RB, DiFrancesco D (1997) Properties and modulation of the I_f current in newborn versus adult cardiac SA node. *Am J Physiol.* **272**:H1549–H1552.

Aimond F, Alvarez JL, Rauzier JM, Lorente P, Vassort G (1999) Ionic basis of ventricular arrhythmias in remodeled rat heart during long-term myocardial infarction. *Cardiovasc Res.* **42**:402–415.

Ambrose JA, Winters SL, Stern A, Eng A, Teichholz LE, Gorlin R, et al (1985) Angiographic evolution of coronary artery morphology and pathogenesis of unstable angina pectoris. *J Am Coll Cardiol.* **5**:609–616.

Anderson JL, Gilbert EM, O'Connell JB, Renland D, Yanowitz K, Murray M, et al (1991) Long-term (2 year) beneficial effects of β-adrenergic blockade with bucindolol in patient with idiopathic dilated cardiomyopathy. *J Am Coll Cardiol.* **17**:1373-1381.

Anderson TJ, Meredith IT, Yeung AC, Frei B, Selwyn AP, Ganz P (1995) The effect of cholesterol-lowering and antioxidant therapy on endothelium dependent coronary vasomotion. *N Engl J Med.* **332**:488–493.

Anzai T, Yoshikawa T, Asakura Y, Abe S, Akaishi M, Mitamura H, et al (1995) Preinfarction angina as a major predictor of left ventricular function and long term prognosis after a first Q wave myocardial infarction. *J Am Coll Cardiol.* **26**:319–327.

Aronow W, Ahn C, Mercando A, Epstein S (1996) Association of average heart rate on 24-hour ambulatory electrocardiograms with incidence of new coronary events at 48-month follow-up in 1,311 patients (mean age 81 years) with heart disease and sinus rhythm. *Am J Cardiol.* **78**:1175–1176.

Aronow WS (1978) Effect of passive smoking on angina pectoris. *N Engl J Med.* **299**:21–24.

Asai K, Uechi M, Sato N, Shen W, Meguro T, Mathier MA, et al (1998) Lack of desensitization and enhanced efficiency of calcium channel promoter in conscious dogs with heart failure. *Am J Physiol.* **275**(6 Pt 2): H2219–2226.

Aupetit JF, Frassati D, Bui-Xuan B, Freysz M, Faucon G, Timour Q (1998) Efficacy of a β-adrenergic receptor antagonist, propranolol, in preventing ischaemic ventricular fibrillation: dependence on heart rate and ischaemia duration. *Cardiovasc Res.* **37**:646–655.

Bahouth SW, Cui X, Beauchamp MJ, Park EA (1997) Thyroid hormone induces beta1-adrenergic receptor gene transcription through a direct repeat separated by five nucleotides. *J Mol Cell Cardiol*, **29**:3223–3237.

Baker K, Warren KS, Yellen G, Fishman MC (1997) Defective "pacemaker" current (I_h) in a zebrafish mutant with a slow heart rate. *Proc Natl Acad Sci U S A.* **94**:4554–4559.

Bauersachs J, Hecker M, Busse R (1994) Display of the characteristics of endothelium-derived hyperpolarizing factor by a cytochrome P450-derived arachidonic acid metabolite in the coronary circulation. *Br J Pharmacol.* **113**:1548–1553.

Beaumont V, Zucker RS (2000) Enhancement of synaptic transmission by cyclic AMP modulation of presynaptic I_h channels. *Nat Neurosci.* **3**:133–141.

Beere PA, Glagov S, Zarins CK (1984) Retarding effect of lowered heart rate on coronary atherosclerosis. *Science.* **226**(4671):180–182.

Beere PA, Glagov S, Zarins CK (1992) Experimental atherosclerosis at the carotid bifurcation of the cynomolgus monkey. Localization, compensatory enlargement, and the sparing effect of lowered heart rate. *Arterioscler Thromb.* **12**:1245–1253.

Bel A, Perrault LP, Faris B, Mouas C, Vilaine J-P, Menasche P (1998) Inhibition of the pacemaker current: a bradycardic therapy for off-pump coronary operations. *Ann Thorac Surg.* **66**:148–152.

Belardinelli L, Giles WR, West A (1988). Ionic mechanisms of adenosine actions in pacemaker cells from rabbit heart. *J Physiol.* **405**:615–633.

Berdeaux A, Drieu La Rochelle C, Richard V, Giudicelli JF (1991) Opposed responses of large and small coronary arteries to propranolol during exercise in dogs. *Am J Physiol.* **261**:H265–H270.

Beuckelmann DJ, Nabauer M, Erdmann E (1993) Alterations of K$^+$ currents in isolated human ventricular myocytes from patients with terminal heart failure. *Circ Res.* **73**:379–385.

Biel M, Zong X, Distler M, Bosse E, Klugbauer N, Murakami M, et al (1994) Another member of the cyclic nucleotide-gated channel family, expressed in testis, kidney, and heart. *Proc Natl Acad Sci U S A.* **91**:3505–3509.

Biel M, Zong X, Ludwig A, Sautter A, Hofmann F (1999) Structure and function of cyclic nucleotide-gated channels. *Rev Physiol Biochem Pharmacol.* **135**:151–171.

Bing OH, Brooks WW, Robinson KG, Slawsky MT, Hayes JA, Litwin SE, et al (1995) The spontaneously hypertensive rat as a model of the transition from compensated left ventricular hypertrophy to failure. *J Mol Cell Cardiol.* **27**:383–396.

Binkley PF, Haas JG, Starling RC, Nunziata E, Hatton PA, Leien CV (1993) Sustained augmentation of parasympathetic tone with angiotensin-converting enzyme inhibition in patients with congestive heart failure. *J Am Coll Cardiol.* **21**:655–661.

Bleeker WK, Mackaay AJC, Masson-Pevet M, Bouman LN, Becker AE (1980) Functional and morphological organization of the rabbit sinus node. *Circ Res.* **46**:11–22.

β-Blocker Heart Attack Trial Research Group (1982) A randomized trial of propranolol in patients with acute myocardial infarction. Mortality results. *JAMA.* **247**:1707–1714.

Bois P, Bescond J, Renaudon B, Lenfant J (1996) Mode of action of bradycardic agent, S 16257, on ionic currents of rabbit sinoatrial node cells. *Br J Pharmacol.* **118**:1051-1057.

Bonaa KH, Arnesen E (1992) Association between heart rate and atherogenic blood lipid fractions in a population. The Tromso Study. *Circulation.* **86**:394–405.

Bonaduce D, Petretta M, Marciano F, Vicario ML, Apicella C, Rao MA, et al (1999) Independent and incremental prognostic value of heart rate variability in patients with chronic heart failure. *Am Heart J.* **138**:273-284.

Borer JS, Fox K, Jaillon P, Lerebours G (2003) Anti-anginal and anti-ischaemic effects of ivbradine, an I_f inhibitor, in stable angina: a randomized, double-blinded, multicenter, placebo-controlled trial. *Circulation.* **107**:817–823.

Bortone AS, Hess OM, Gaglione A, Suter T, Nonogi H, Grimm J, et al (1990) Effect of propranolol on coronary vasomotion in response to sympathetic stimulation in humans: importance of the functional integrity of the endothelium. *Circulation.* **81**:1225–1235.

Boskabady MH, Snashall PD (2000) Bronchial responsiveness to beta-adrenergic stimulation and enhanced beta-blockade in asthma. *Respirology.* **5**:111–118.

BoSmith RE, Briggs I, Sturgess NC (1993) Inhibitory actions of ZENECA ZD7288 on whole-cell hyperpolarization activated inward current (I_f) in guinea-pig dissociated sinoatrial node cells. *Br J Pharmacol.* **110**:343–349.

Bristow MR (2000) β-Adrenergic receptor blockade in chronic heart failure. *Circulation.* **101**:558–569.

Bristow MR, Ginsburg R, Minobe W, Cubicciotti RS, Sageman WS, Lurie K, et al (1982) Decreased catecholamine sensitivity and β-adrenergic-receptor density in failing human hearts. *N Engl J Med.* **307**:205-211.

Bristow MR, Ginsburg R, Umans V, Fowler M, Minobe W, Rasmussen R, et al (1986) β1- and β2-adrenergic-receptor subpopulations in nonfailing and failing human ventricular myocardium: coupling of both receptor subtypes to muscle contraction and selective beta 1-receptor downregulation in heart failure. *Circ Res.* **59**:297–309.

Brochu RM, Clay JR, Shrier A (1992) Pacemaker current in single cells and in aggregates of cells dissociated from the embryonic chick heart. *J Physiol (Lond.)* **454**:503–515.

Brouwer J, van Veldhuisen DJ, Man in 't Veld AJ, Dunselman PH, Broomsma F, Haaksma J, et al (1995) Heart rate variability in patients with mild to moderate heart failure: effect of neurohormonal modulation by digoxin and ibopamine multicenter trial (DIMT) study group. *J Am Coll Cardiol.* **26**:983-990.

Brouwer J, Van Veldhuisen DJ, Man In 't Veld AJ (1996) Prognostic value of heart rate variability during long term follow-up in patients with mild to moderate heart failure. *J Am Coll Cardiol.* **28**:1183–1189.

Brown HF, DiFrancesco D (1980) Voltage clamp investigations of membrane currents underlying pacemaker activity in rabbit sino-atrial node. *J Physiol.* **308**:331–351.

Brown HF, DiFrancesco D, Noble SJ (1979) How does adrenaline accelerate the heart? *Nature.* **280**:235–236.

Browne DL, Gancher ST, Nutt JG, Brunt ER, Smith EA, Kramer P, et al (1994) Episodic ataxia/myokymia syndrome is associated with point mutations in the human potassium channel gene, KCNA1. *Nat Genet.* **8**:136–140.

Bucchi A, Baruscotti M, DiFrancesco D (2002) Current-dependent block of rabbit sino-atrial node I_f channels by ivabradine. *J Gen Physiol.* **120**:1–13.

Burke AP, Farb A, Malcom GT, You-hui Liang, Smialek J, Virmani R (1997) Coronary risk factors and plaque morphology in men with coronary disease who died suddenly. *N Engl J Med.* **336**:1276–1282.

Campbell J, King SB, Douglas JS, et al (1985): Prevalence and distribution of disease in patients catheterized for suspected coronary disease. In: King SB, Douglas JS (eds.) *Coronary arteriography and angioplasty.* New York, NY: McGraw Hill; p 365.

Casolo G, Balli E, Taddei T, Amusasi J, Gori C (1989) Decreased spontaneous heart rate variability in congestive heart failure. *Am J Cardiol.* **64**:1162–1167.

Castellano M, Bohm M (1997) The cardiac β-adrenoceptor-mediated signaling pathway and its alterations in hypertensive heart disease. *Hypertension.* **29**:715–722.

Castelli WP, Levy D, Wilson PWF, Kannel W (1990) Sudden death: the view from Framingham. In: Kostis JB, Sanders M, (eds). *The prevention of sudden death.* New York, NY: E Wiley-Liss; pp 1-8.

Cerbai E, Barbieri M, Li Q, Mugelli A (1994a) Ionic basis of action potential prolongation of hypertrophied cardiac myocytes isolated from hypertensive rats of different ages. *Cardiovasc Res.* **28**:1180–1187.

Cerbai E, Barbieri M, Mugelli A (1994b) Characterization of the hyperpolarization-activated current, I(f), in ventricular myocytes isolated from hypertensive rats. *J Physiol.* **481**:585–591.

Cerbai E, Barbieri M, Mugelli A (1996) Occurrence and properties of the hyperpolarization-activated current I_f in ventricular myocytes from normotensive and hypertensive rats during aging. *Circulation.* **94**:1674–1681.

Cerbai E, Barbieri M, Porciatti F, Mugelli A (1995) Ionic channels in hypertrophy and heart failure: relevance for arrhythmogenesis. *New Trends Arrhythmias.* **11**:135–139.

Cerbai E, Crucitti A, Sartiani L, De Paoli P, Pino R, Rodriguez ML, et al (2000) Long-term treatment of spontaneously hypertensive rats with losartan and electrophysiological remodeling of cardiac myocytes. *Cardiovasc Res.* **45**:388–396.

Cerbai E, Pino R, Porciatti F, Sani G, Toscano M, Maccherini M, et al (1997) Characterization of the hyperpolarization-activated current, I_f, in ventricular myocytes from human failing heart. *Circulation.* **95**:568–571.

Cerbai E, Pino R, Rodriguez ML, Mugelli A (1999a) Modulation of the pacemaker current I_f by β-adrenoceptor subtypes in ventricular myocytes isolated from hypertensive and normotensive rats. *Cardiovasc Res.* **42**:121–129.

Cerbai E, Pino R, Sartiani L, Mugelli A (1999b) Influence of postnatal-development on I_f occurrence and properties in neonatal rat ventricular myocytes. *Cardiovasc Res.* **42**:416–423.

Cerbai E, Sartiani L, DePaoli P, Pino R, Maccherini M, Bizzarri F, et al (2001) The properties of the pacemaker current I_f in human ventricular myocytes are modulated by cardiac disease. *J Mol Cell Cardiol.* **33**:441–448.

Cerbai E, Zaza A, Mugelli A (1999c) Pharmacology of membrane ion channels in human myocytes. In: Zipes D, Jalife, (eds) *Cardiac Electrophysiology: From Cell to Bedside*, 3rd ed, Philadephia, Penn: WB Saunders Co; 167–173.

Chandra R, Herweg B, Rosen TS, Danilo P Jr, Rosen MR (2000) Altered activation induces atrial memory and atrial tachyarrhythmias in canine heart. *Circulation.* **102**:1579. (Abstract)

Chang F, Cohen IS, DiFrancesco D, Rosen MR, Tromba C (1991) Effects of protein kinase inhibitors on canine purkinje fibre pacemaker depolarization and the pacemaker current I_f. *J Physiol.* **440**:367–384.

Chang F, Yu H, Cohen IS (1994) Actions of vasoactive intestinal peptide and neuropeptide Y on the pacemaker current in canine Purkinje fibers. *Circ Res.* **74**:157–162.

Chen J, Mitcheson JS, Lin M, Sanguinetti MC (2000) Functional roles of charged residues in the putative voltage sensor of the HCN2 pacemaker channel. *J Biol Chem.* **275**:36465–36471.

Chen W, Gabel S, Steenbergen S, Murphy E (1995) A redox based mechanism of cardiac protection induced by ischemic pre-conditioning in perfused rat heart. *Circ Res.* **77**:424–429.

Chen, RY, Fan FC, Schuessler GB, Chien S (1982) Baroreflex control of heart rate in humans during nitroprusside-induced hypotension. *Am J Physiol.* **243**:R18–R24.

Chiamvimonat V, Newman D, Tang A, Green M, Mitchell J, Wulffhart Z, et al (1998) A double-blind placebo-controlled evaluation of the human electrophysiologic effects of zatebradine, a sinus node inhibitor. *J Cardiovasc Pharmacol.* **32**:516–520.

Chien KR (1999) Stress pathways and heart failure. *Cell.* **98**:555–558.

CIBIS II Investigators and Committees (1999) The Cardiac Insufficiency Bisoprolol Study II (CIBIS II): a randomized trial. *Lancet.* **353**:9–13.

CIBIS Investigators and Committees (1994) A randomized trial of β-blockade in heart failure: the cardiac insufficiency bisoprolol study (CIBIS). *Circulation.* **90**:1765-1773.

Clapham DE (1998) Not so funny anymore: pacing channels are cloned. *Neuron.* **21**:5–7.

Clay JR, De Haan RL (1979) Fluctuations in interbeat interval in rhythmic heart cells clusters. *Biophys J.* **28**:377–390.

Conway J (1984) Hemodynamic aspects of essential hypertension in humans. *Physiol Rev.* **64**:617–660.

Copie X, Hnatkova H, Staunton A, Fei L, Camm AJ, Malik M (1996a) Predictive power of increased heart rate versus depressed left ventricular ejection fraction and heart rate variability for risk stratification after myocardial infarction. Results of a two year follow-up study. *J Am Coll Cardiol.* **27**:270–276.

Copie X, Le Heuzey JY, Iliou MC, Lavergne T, Guize L (1996b) Correlation between time-domain measures of heart rate variability and scatterplots in post infarction patients. *Pacing Clin Electrophysiol.* **19**:342–347.

Copie X, Pousset F, Lechat P, Jaillon P, Guize L, Le Heuzey JY (1996c) Effects of beta-blockade with bisoprolol on heart rate variability in advanced heart failure: analysis of scatterplots of RR intervals at selected heart rate. *Am Heart J.* **132**:369–375.

Costard-Jäckle A, Goetsch B, Antz M, Franz MR (1989) Slow and long-lasting modulation of myocardial repolarization produced by ectopic activation in isolated rabbit hearts. Evidence for cardiac "memory". *Circulation.* **80**:1412–1420.

Davies CH, Davia K, Bennett JG, Pepper JR, Poole-Wilson PA, Harding SE (1995) Reduced contraction and altered frequency response of isolated ventricular myocytes from patients with heart failure. *Circulation.* **92**:2540–2549.

de Rooij J, Zwartkruis FJ, Verheijen MH, Cool RH, Nijman SM, Wittinghofer A, et al (1998) Epac is a Rap1 guanine-nucleotide exchange factor directly activated by cyclic AMP. *Nature.* **396**:474–477.

del Balzo U, Rosen MR (1992) T wave changes persisting after ventricular pacing in canine heart are altered by 4-aminopyridine but not by lidocaine. *Circulation.* **85**:1464–1472.

Delfaut P, Saksena S, Prakash A, Krol RB (1998) Long-term outcome of patients with drug-refractory atrial flutter and fibrillation after single- and dual-site right atrial pacing for arrhythmia prevention. *J Am Coll Cardiol.* **32**:1900–1908.

Demontis GC, Longoni B, Barcaro U, Cervetto L (1999) Properties and functional roles of hyperpolarization-gated currents in guinea-pig retinal rods. *J Physiol.* **515**:813–828.

Denyer JC, Brown HF (1990) Pacemaking in rabbit isolated sino-atrial node cells during Cs^+ block of the hyperpolarization-activated current I_f. *J Physiol.* **429**:401–409.

Di Carli MF, Maddahi J, Rokhsar S, Schelbert HR, Bianco-Batlles D, Brunken RC, et al (1998) Long-term survival of patients with coronary artery disease and left ventricular dysfunction: implications for the role of myocardial viability assessment in management decisions. *J Thorac Cardiovasc Surg.* **116**:997–1004.

DiFrancesco D (1981a) A new interpretation of the pacemaker current in calf Purkinje fibres. *J Physiol.* **314**:359–376.

DiFrancesco D (1981b) A study of the ionic nature of the pacemaker current in calf Purkinje fibres. *J Physiol.* **314**:377–393.

DiFrancesco D (1982) Block and activation of the pacemaker I_f channel in calf Purkinje fibres: effects of potassium, caesium and rubidium. *J Physiol.* **329**:485–507.

DiFrancesco D (1985) The cardiac hyperpolarizing-activated current I_f. Origins and development. *Prog Biophys Mol Biol.* **46**:163–183.

DiFrancesco D (1986) Characterization of single pacemaker channels in cardiac sino-atrial node cells. *Nature.* **324**:470–473.

DiFrancesco D (1991) The contribution of the "pacemaker" current (I_f) to generation of spontaneous activity in rabbit sino-atrial node myocytes. *J Physiol.* **434**:23–40.

DiFrancesco D (1993) Pacemaker mechanisms in cardiac tissue. *Annu Rev Physiol.* **55**:455–472.

DiFrancesco D (1994) Some properties of the UL-FS 49 block of the hyperpolarization-activated (I_f) current in SA node myocytes. *Pflügers Arch.* **427**:64–70.

DiFrancesco D (1995a) The pacemaker current (I_f) plays an important role in regulating SA node pacemaker activity. *Cardiovasc Res.* **30**:307-308

DiFrancesco D (1995b) The onset and autonomic regulation of cardiac pacemaker activity: relevance of the I_f current. *Cardiovasc Res.* **29**:449–456.

DiFrancesco D, Ducouret P, Robinson RB (1989) Muscarinic modulation of cardiac rate at low acetylcholine concentrations. *Science.* **243**:669–671.

DiFrancesco D, Ferroni A, Mazzanti M, Tromba C (1986) Properties of the hyperpolarizing-activated current (I_f) in cells isolated from the rabbit sino-atrial node. *J Physiol.* **377**:61–88.

DiFrancesco D, Mangoni M (1994) The modulation of single hyperpolarization-activated (I_f) channels by cyclic AMP in the rabbit SA node. *J Physiol.* **474**:473–482.

DiFrancesco D, Noble D (1989) Current I_f and its contribution to cardiac pacemaking. In: Jacklet JW (ed.) *Neuronal and cellular oscillators.* New York, NY: Dekker; 31–57.

DiFrancesco D, Tortora P (1991) Direct activation of cardiac pacemaker channels by intracellular cyclic AMP. *Nature.* **351**:145–147.

DiFrancesco D, Tromba C (1987) Acetylcholine inhibits activation of the cardiac hyperpolarizing-activated current I_f. *Pflügers Arch.* **410**:139-142.

DiFrancesco D, Tromba C (1988) Muscarinic control of the hyperpolarizing-activated current I_f in rabbit sino-atrial node myocytes. *J Physiol.* **405**:493–510.

Doerr T, Trautwein W (1990) On the mechanism of the "specific bradycardic action" of the verapamil derivative UL-FS 49. *Naunyn Schmiedebergs Arch Pharmacol.* **341**:331–340.

Doyle DA, Cabral JM, Pfuetzner RA, Kuo A, Gulbis JM, Cohen SL, et al (1998) The structure of the potassium channel: molecular basis of K⁺ conduction and selectivity. *Science.* **280**:69–77.

Dyer AR, Persky V, Stamler J, Paul O, Shekelle RB, Berkson DM, et al (1980) Heart rate as a prognostic factor for coronary heart disease and mortality: findings in three Chicago epidemiologic studies. *Am J Epidemiol.* **112**:736–749.

Egstrup K (1988) Transient myocardial ischemia after abrupt withdrawal of antianginal therapy in chronic stable angina. *Am J Cardiol.* **61**:1219–1222.

Eliot R, Buell JC (1985) Role of emotions and stress in the genesis of sudden death. *J Am Coll Cardiol.* **5**:95B–98B.

Ewing DJ, Campbell IW, Clarke BF (1981) Heart rate changes in diabetes mellitus. *Lancet.* **1**:183–185.

Fain GL, Quandt FN, Bastian BL (1978) Contribution of a cesium-sensitive conductance increase to the rod photoresponse. *Nature.* **272**:467–469.

Falk E, Shah PK, Fuster V (1995) Coronary plaque disruption. *Circulation.* **92**:657–671.

Faplan AD, Goodfield NE, Wright RA, Francis CM, Neilson JM (1997) Effect of digoxin on time domain measures of heart rate variability in patients with stable chronic cardiac failure: withdrawal and comparison group studies. *Int J Cardiol.* **59**:29-36.

Farès N, Bois P, Lenfant J, Potreau D (1998) Characterization of a hyperpolarization-activated current in dedifferentiated adult ventricular cells in primary culture. *J Physiol.* **506**:73–82.

Feldman MD, Alderman JD, Aroesty JM, Royal HD, Ferguson JJ, Owen RM, et al (1988) Depression of systolic and diastolic myocardial reserve during atrial pacing tachycardia in patients with dilated cardiomyopathy. *J Clin Invest.* **82**:1661-1669.

Fihn SD, Williams SV, Daley J, Gibbons RJ, American College of Cardiology, American Heart Association, American College of Physicians-American Society of Internal Medicine (2001) Guidelines for the management of patients with chronic stable angina: treatment. *Ann Intern Med.* **135**:616–632.

Floras JS (1993) Clinical aspects of sympathetic activation and parasympathetic withdrawal in heart failure. *J Am Coll Cardiol.* **22(A)**: 72-84.

Foster AH, Geld MR, McLaughlin JS (1995) Acute hemodynamic effects of atrio-biventricular pacing in humans. *Ann Thorac Surg.* **59**:294–300.

Fowler MB, Laser JA, Hopkins GL, Minobe W, Bristow MR (1986) Assessment of the beta-adrenergic receptor pathway in the intact failing human heart: progressive β-receptor down-regulation and specific pharmacologic subsensitivity to agonist response. *Circulation.* **74**:1290-1302.

Frace AM, Maruoka F, Noma A (1992a) External K$^+$ increases Na$^+$ conductances of the hyperpolarization-activated current in rabbit cardiac pacemaker cells. *Pflügers Arch.* **421**:94–96.

Frace AM, Maruoka F, Noma A (1992b) Control of the hyperpolarization-activated cation current by external anions in rabbit sino-atrial node cells. *J Physiol.* **453**:307–318.

Freudenberg H, Lichtlen PR (1981) The normal wall segment in coronary stenosis: a post mortem study. *Z Kardiol.* **70**:863–869.

Fujita M, Miyamoto S, Sekiguchi H, Eiho S, Sasayama S (2000) Effects of posture on sympathetic nervous modulation in patients with chronic heart failure. *Lancet.* **356**:1822-1823.

Fujiura Y, Adachi H, Tsuruta M, Jacobs DR Jr, Hirai Y, Imaizumi T (2001) Heart rate and mortality in a Japanese general population: an 18-year follow-up study. *J Clin Epidemiol.* **54**: 495–500.

Furchgott RF, Zawadski JV (1980) The obligatory role of endothelial cells in the relaxation of arterial smooth muscle cells by acetylcholine. *Nature.* **288**:373–376.

Gadler F, Linde C, Juhlin-Dannfelt A, Ribeiro A, Ryden L (1997) Long-term effects of dual chamber pacing in patients with hypertrophic obstructive cardiomyopathy without outflow obstruction at rest. *Eur Heart J.* **18**:636–642.

Ganz W, Watanabe I, Kanamas K (1990) Does reperfusion extend necrosis? A study in a single territory of myocardial ischemia–half reperfused and half not reperfused. *Circulation.* **82**:1020–1033.

Gardiner SM, Kemp PA, March JE, Bennett T (1995) Acute and chronic cardiac and regional haemodynamic effects of the novel bradycardic agent, S16257, in conscious rats. *Br J Pharmacol.* **115**:579-586.

Gasparini S, DiFrancesco D (1997) Action of the hyperpolarization-activated (I_h) current blocker ZD 7288 in hippocampal CA1 neurons. *Pflügers Arch.* **435**:99–106.

Gauss R, Deifert R, Kaupp UB (1998) Molecular identification of a hyperpolarization-activated channel in sea urchin sperm. *Nature.* **393**:583–587.

Gerdes AM, Onodera T, Wang X, McCune SA (1996) Myocyte remodeling during the progression to failure in rats with hypertension. *Hypertension.* **28**:609–614.

Gibbons RJ, Chatterjee K, Daley J, Douglas JS, Fihn SD, Gardin JM, et al (1999) ACC/AHA/ACP–ASIM guidelines for the management of patients with chronic stable angina: executive summary and recommendations. A report of the American College of Cardiology/American Heart Association Task Force on Practice Guidelines (Committee on Management of patients with Chronic Stable Angina). *Circulation.* **99**:2829–2848.

Gilbert EM, Anderson JL, Deitchman D, Yanowitz FG, O'Connell JB, Renlund DG, et al (1990) Long-term β-blocker-vasodilator therapy improves cardiac function in idiopathic dilated cardiomyopathy: a double-blind, randomized study of bucindolol versus placebo. *Am J Med.* **88**:223-239.

Gillman M, Kannel W, Belanger A, D'Agostino R (1993) Influence of heart rate on mortality among persons with hypertension: The Framingham study. *Am Heart J.* **125**:1148–1154.

Gillum R (1988) The epidemiology of resting heart rate in a national sample of men and women: Association with hypertension, coronary heart disease, blood pressure, and other cardiovascular risk factors. *Am Heart J.* **116**:163–174.

Gillum R, Makuc D, Feldman J (1991) Pulse rate, coronary heart disease, and death: The NHANES I epidemiologic follow-up study. *Am Heart J.* **121**:172–177.

Gloss B, Trost SU, Bluhm WF, Swanson EA, Clark R, Winkfein KM, et al (2001) Cardiac ion channel expression and contractile function in mice with deletion of thyroid hormone receptor α or β. *Endocrinology.* **142**:544–550.

Goethals M, Raes A, Van Bogaert PP (1993) Use-dependent block of the pacemaker current I_f in rabbit sino-atrial node cells by zatebradine (UL-FS49). On the mode of action of sinus node inhibitors. *Circulation.* **88**:2389-2401.

Goldberg R, Larson M, Levy D (1996) Factors associated with survival to 75 years of age in middle-aged men and women: The Framingham study. *Arch Intern Med.* **156**:505–509.

Gould KL (1985) Quantification of coronary artery stenosis in vivo. *Circ Res.* **57**:341–353.

Gould KL, Lipscomb K, Hamilton GW (1974) Physiologic basis for assessing critical coronary stenosis: instantaneous flow response and regional distribution during coronary hyperemia as a measure of coronary flow reserve. *Am J Cardiol.* **33**:87–94.

Goulding EH, Tibbs GR, Siegelbaum SA (1994) Molecular mechanism of cyclic nucleotide-gated channel activation. *Nature.* **372**:369–374.

Green M, Peled I (1992) Prevalence and control of hypertension in a large cohort of occupationally-active Israelis examined during 1985–1987. The CORDIS Study. *Int J Epidemiol.* **21**:674–682.

Gross G, Auchampach JA (1992) Blockade of ATP-sensitive potassium channels prevents myocardial pre-conditioning in dogs. *Circ Res.* **70**:223–233.

Gundersen T, Grottum P, Pedersen T, Kjekshus J, for the Norwegian Timolol Multi-center Study Group (1986) Effect of timolol on mortality and reinfarction after acute myocardial infarction: Prognostic importance of heart rate at rest. *Am J Cardiol.* **58**:20–24.

Guo W, Kamiya K, Hojo M, Kodama I, Toyama J (1998) Regulation of Kv4.2 and Kv1.4 K$^+$ channel expression by myocardial hypertrophic factors in cultured newborn rat ventricular cells. *J Mol Cell Cardiol.* **30**:1449–1455.

Guo W, Kamiya K, Toyama J (1996) Modulated expression of transient outward current in cultured neonatal rat ventricular myocytes: comparison with development in situ. *Cardiovasc Res.* **32**:524–533.

Guth BD, Dietze T (1995) I_f current mediates beta-adrenergic enhancement of heart rate but not contractility in vivo. *Bas Res Cardiol.* **90**:192-202.

Gwathmey JK, Copelas L, MacKinnon R (1987) Abnormal intracellular calcium handling in myocardium from patients with end-stage heart failure. *Circ Res.* **61**:70-76.

Gwathmey JK, Slawsky MT, Hajjar RJ (1990) Role of intracellular calcium handling in force-interval relationships of human ventricular myocardium. *J Clin Invest.* **85**:1599-1613.

Habib G (1997) Reappraisal of the importance of heart rate as a risk factor for cardiovascular morbidity and mortality. *Clin Therapeut.* **19(Suppl A)**:39–55.

Habib G (2001) Is heart rate a risk factor in the general population? *Dialogues in Cardiovascular Medicine.* **6**:25–31.

Hakamaki T, Lehtonen A (1997) Metabolic effects of spirapril and atenolol: results from a randomized, long-term study. *Int J Clin Pharmacol Ther.* **35**:227–230.

Hallstrom AP, Cobb LA, Yu BH, Weaver WD, Fahrenbruch CE (1991) An antiarrhythmic drug experience in 941 patients resuscitated from an initial cardiac arrest between 1970 and 1985. *Am J Cardiol.* **68**:1025–1031.

Hamer AWF, Arkles LB, Johns JA (1989) Beneficial effects of low dose amiodarone in patients with congestive heart failure: a placebo controlled trial. *J Am Coll Cardiol.* **14**:1768-1174.

Harrison DG (1996) Endothelial control of vasomotion and nitric oxide production. *Cardiology Clinics.* **14**:1–15.

Hasenfuss G, Holubarsch C, Hermann HP, Astheimer K, Pieshe B, Just H (1994) Influence of the force-frequency relationship on haemodynamics and left ventricular function in patients with dilated cardiomiopathy. *Eur Heart J.* **15**:164-170.

Hayashi H, Okajima M, Yamada K (1976a) Atrial T (Ta) loop in dogs with or without atrial injury. *Am Heart J.* **91**:607–617.

Hayashi H, Okajima M, Yamada K (1976b) Atrial T (Ta) loop in patients with A-V block: A trial to differentiate normal and abnormal groups. *Am Heart J.* **91**:491–500.

Heginbotham L, Lu Z, Abramson T, MacKinnon R (1994) Mutations in the K^+ channel signature sequence. *Biophys J.* **66**:1061–1067.

Heidenreich PA, Lee TT, Massie BM (1997) Effect of β-blockade on mortality in patients with heart failure: a meta-analysis of randomized clinical trial. *J Am Coll Cardiol.* **30**:27-34.

Heilbrunn SM, Shah P, Bristow MR, Valentine HA, Ginsbury R, Fowler MB (1989) Increased β-receptor density and improved haemodynamic response to catecholamine stimulation during long-term metoprolol therapy in heart failure from dilated cardiomyopathy. *Circulation.* **79**:483-490.

Hermann HP, Ohler A, Just H, Hasenfuss G (1998) Cardiac and haemodynamic effect of the sinus node inhibitor tedisamil dihidrochloride in patients with congestive heart failure due to dilated cardiomyopathy. *J Cardiovasc Pharmacol.* **32**:969-974.

Herweg B, Chang F, Chandra P, Danilo P Jr, Rosen MR (2001) Cardiac memory in canine atrium. Identification and implications. *Circulation.* **103**:455–461.

Hinkle L Jr (1981) The immediate antecedents of sudden death. *Acta Med Scand.* **651**:207–217.

Hittinger L, Shannon RP, Bishop SP, Gelpi RJ, Vatner SF (1989) Subendomyocardial exhaustion of blood flow reserve and increased fibrosis in conscious dogs with heart failure. *Circ Res.* **65**:971–980.

Hjalmarson A (1990) Heart rate and β-adrenergic mechanisms in acute myocardial infarction. *Basic Res Cardiol.* **85**:325–333.

Hjalmarson A (1997) Effects of β blockade on sudden cardiac death during acute myocardial infarction and the postinfarction period. *Am J Cardiol.* **80**(9B):35J–39J.

Hjalmarson A, Gilpin EA, Kjekshus J, Schieman G, Nicod P, Henning H, et al (1990) Influence of heart rate on mortality after acute myocardial infarction. *Am J Cardiol.* **65**:547–553.

Ho WK, Brown HF, Noble D (1994) High selectivity of the I_f channels to Na^+ and K^+ in rabbit isolated sinoatrial node cells. *Pflügers Arch.* **426**:68–74.

Homcy CJ, Vatner SF, Vatner DE (1991) β-adrenergic receptor regulation in the heart in pathophysiologic states: abnormal adrenergic responsiveness in cardiac disease. *Annu Rev Physiol.* **53**:137–159.

Hoppe UC, Jansen E, Südkamp M, Beuckelmann DJ (1998) Hyperpolarization-activated inward current in ventricular myocytes from normal and failing human hearts. *Circulation.* **97**:55–65.

Irisawa H, Brown HF, Giles W (1993) Cardiac pacemaking in the sinoatrial node. *Physiol Rev.* **73**:197–227.

Ishii TM, Takano M, Xie LH, Noma A, Ohmori H (1999) Molecular characterization of the hyperpolarization-activated cation channel in rabbit heart sinoatrial node. *J Biol Chem.* **274**:12835–12839.

Isner JM, Walsh K, Symes J, Pieczek A, Takeshita S, Lowry J, et al (1995) Arterial gene therapy for therapeutic angiogenesis in patients with peripheral artery disease. *Circulation.* **91**:2687–2692.

James RG, Arnold JM, Allen JD, Pantridge JF, Shanks RG (1977) The effects of heart rate, myocardial ischemia and vagal stimulation on the threshold for ventricular fibrillation. *Circulation.* **55**:311–317.

Janse MJ, Wit AL (1989) Electrophysiologic mechanisms of ventricular arrhythmias resulting from myocardial ischemia and infarction. *Physiol Rev.* **69**:1049–1152.

Jessup M (1991) Beta-adrenergic blockade in congestive heart failure: answering the old questions. *J Am Coll Cardiol.* **18**:1067–1069.

Julian DG, Prescott RJ, Jackson FS, Szekely P (1982) Controlled trial of sotalol for one year after myocardial infarction. *Lancet.* **1**(8282):1142–1147.

Julius S (1993) Sympathetic hyperactivity and coronary artery risk in hypertension. *Hypertension.* **21**:886–891.

Kanazawa T (1994) Coronary collateral circulation—its development and function. *Jpn Circ J.* **58**:151–165.

Kaneko A, Tachibana M (1985) A voltage-clamp analysis of membrane currents in solitary bipolar cells dissociated from *Carassius aureus. J Physiol.* **358**:131–152.

Kannel W, Wilson P, Blaire S (1985) Epidemiologic assessment of the role of physical activity and fitness in development of cardiovascular disease. *Am Heart J.* **109**:876–885.

Kannel WB, Kannel C, Paffenbarger RS Jr, Cupples LA (1987) Heart rate and cardiovascular mortality: the Framingham Study. *Am Heart J.* **113**:1489–1494.

Kaplan JR, Manuck SB, Adams MR, Weingand KW, Clarkson TB (1987b) Inhibition of coronary atherosclerosis by propranolol in behaviorally predisposed monkeys fed an atherogenic diet. *Circulation.* **76**:1364–1372.

Kaplan JR, Manuck SB, Clarkson TB (1987a) The influence of heart rate on coronary artery atherosclerosis. *J Cardiovasc Pharmacol.* **10(Suppl 2)**: S100–S102; discussion S103.

Kaplan JR, Manuck SB, Clarkson TB, Lusso FM, Taub DM (1982) Social status, environment and atherosclerosis in cynomolgus monkeys. *Arteriosclerosis.* **2**:359–368.

Katz AM (1992) T wave "memory": possible causal relationship to stress-induced changes in cardiac ion channels? *J Cardiovasc Electrophysiol.* **3**:150–159.

Kaupp UB, Seifert R (2001) Molecular diversity of pacemaker ion channels. *Annu Rev Physiol.* **63**:235–257.

Kawasaki H, Springett GM, Mochizuki N, Toki S, Nakaya M, Matsuda M, *et al* (1998) A family of cAMP-binding proteins that directly activate Rap1. *Science.* **282**:2275–2279.

Kendall MJ, Lynch KP, Hjalmarson A, Kjekshus J (1995) β-blockers and sudden cardiac death. *Ann Intern Med.* **123**:358–367.

Kilborn MJ, Fedida D (1990) A study of the developmental changes in outward currents of rat ventricular myocytes. *J Physiol (Lond.).* **430**:37–60.

Kjekshus J (1985) Comments—β-blockers: Heart rate reduction a mechanism of benefit. *Eur Heart J.* **6**:29–30.

Kjekshus J (1986) Importance of heart rate in determining β-blocker efficacy in acute and long-term acute myocardial infarction intervention trials. *Am J Cardiol.* **57**:43F–49F.

Kleiger RE, Miller JP, Bigger JT, Moss AJ (1987) Decreased heart rate variability and its association with increased mortality after acute myocardial infarction. *Am J Cardiol.* **59**:256–262.

Klein I, Ojamaa K (1998) Thyrotoxicosis and the heart. *Thyrotoxicosis.* **27**:51–62.

Kobinger W, Lillie C (1987) Specific bradycardic agents—a novel pharmacological class? *Eur Heart J.* **8**:7–15.

Konstam MA, Remme WJ (1998) Treatment guidelines in heart failure. *Prog Cardiovasc Dis.* **41**:65–72.

Kristal-Boneh E, Silber H, Harari G, Froom P (2000) The association of resting heart rate with cardiovascular, cancer and all-cause mortality. Eight-year follow-up of 3527 male Israeli employees (the CORDIS Study). *Eur Heart J.* **21**:16–124.

Krone W, Nagele H (1988) Effects of antihypertensives on plasma lipids and lipoprotein metabolism. *Am Heart J.* **116**:1729–1734.

Krum H, Bigger JT, Goldsmith RL, Packer M (1995) Effects of long-term digoxin therapy on autonomic function in patients with chronic heart failure. *J Am Coll Cardiol.* **25**:289–294.

Le Heuzey JY, Guize L, Moutet JP, Cabanis C, Maurice P, Peronneau P (1982) Intra SA nodal pacemaker shift: indirect evaluation in the open chest dog. *Cardiovasc Res.* **16**:276–282.

Le Heuzey JY, Guize L, Valty J, Lavergne T, Moutet JP, Peronneau P (1986) Intracellular and extracellular recordings of sinus node activation: comparison with estimated sino atrial conduction time during pacemaker shift in rabbit heart. *Cardiovasc Res.* **20**:81–88.

Lechat PP, Packer M, Chalon S (1998) Clinical effects of β-adrenergic blockade in chronic heart failure: a meta-analysis of double blind, placebo-controlled randomised trial. *Circulation.* **98**:1184-1191.

Leenen FHH (1999) Cardiovascular consequences of sympathetic hyperactivity. *Can J Cardiol.* **15(Suppl A)**:2A–12A.

Lerman A, Burnett JC JR (1992) Intact and altered endothelium in regulation of vasomotion. *Circulation.* **86**:12–19.

Levy D, Larson MG, Basal RS, Kannel WB, Ho KL (1996) The progression from hypertension to congestive heart failure. *JAMA.* **275**:1557–1562.

Lewis RV, Lofthouse C (1993) Adverse reactions with beta-adrenoceptor blocking drugs. An update. *Drug Saf.* **4**:272–279.

Lillie C, Singh BN (1994) Sinus Node Inhibitors. In: Singh BN, Dzau VJ, Vanhoutte PM, Woosley RL (eds). *Cardiovascular Pharmacology and Therapeutics.* New York, NY: Churchill Livingstone; pp 203–216.

Lithell H, Pollare T, Vessby B (1992) Metabolic effects of pindolol and propranolol in a double-blind crossover study in hypertensive patients. *Blood Press.* **1**:92–101.

Littleton JT, Ganetzky B (2000) Ion channels and synaptic organization: analysis of the *Drosophila* genome. *Neuron.* **26**:35–43.

Ludmer P, Selwyn AP, Shook TL, Wayne RR, Mudge GH, Alexander RW, *et al* (1986) Paradoxical vasoconstriction induced by acetylcholine in atherosclerotic coronary arteries. *N Engl J Med.* **315**:1046–1051.

Ludwig A, Zong X, Hofmann F, Biel M (1999a) Structure and function of cardiac pacemaker channels. *Cell Physiol Biochem.* **9**:179–186.

Ludwig A, Zong X, Jeglitsch M, Hofmann F, Biel M (1998) A family of hyperpolarization-activated mammalian cation channels. *Nature*. **393**:587–591.

Ludwig A, Zong X, Stieber J, Hullin R, Hofmann F, Biel M (1999b) Two pacemaker channels from human heart with profoundly different activation kinetics. *EMBO J*. **18**:2323–2329.

Lundberg JM, Hökfelt T (1986) Multiple co-existence of peptides and classical transmitters in peripheral autonomic and sensory neurons: functional and pharmacological implications. *Prog Brain Res*. **68**:241–262.

Lux RL, Urie PM, Burgess MJ, Abildskov JA (1980) Variability of the body surface distribution of QRS, ST-T and QRST deflection areas with varied activation sequence in dogs. *Cardiovasc Res*. **14**:607–612.

Magee JC (1999) Dendritic I_h normalizes temporal summation in hippocampus CA1 neurons. *Nat Neurosci*. **18**:7613–7624.

Malik M (1995) Geometrical methods for heart rate variability assessment. In: Malik M, Camm AJ, (eds.) *Heart rate variability*. New York, NY: Futura Publishing Co; 47–62.

Management of stable angina pectoris. Recommendations of the Task Force of the European Society of Cardiology. *Eur Heart J* 1997;**18**:394–413.

Mangin L, Swynghedauw B, Benis A, Thibault N, Lerebours G, Carre F (1998) Relationship between heart rate and heart rate variability: study in conscious rats. *J Cardiovasc Pharmacol*. **32**:601-607.

Mangoni AA, Mircoli L, Giannattasib C, Ferrari AU, Mancia G (1996) Heart rate-dependence of arterial distensibility in vivo. *J Hypertens*. **14**:897–901.

Manuck SB, Kaplan JR, Clarkson TB (1986) Atherosclerosis, social dominance, and cardiovascular reactivity. In: Schmidt TH, Dembroski TM, Blumchen G, (eds.) *Biological and psychological factors in cardiovascular disease*. Berlin, Heidelberg, Germany: Springer-Verlag; 459–475.

Marban E (1991) Myocardial stunning and hibernation: the physiology behind the colloquialisms. *Circulation*. **83**:681–688.

Maroko PR, Kjekshus JK, Sobel BE, Watanabe T, Covell JW, Ross J Jr, et al (1971) Factors influencing infarct size following experimental coronary artery occlusions. *Circulation*. **43**:67–82.

Mayer ML, Westbrook GL (1983) A voltage-clamp analysis of inward (anomalous) rectification in mouse spinal sensory ganglion neurones. *J Physiol*. **340**:19–45.

McCormick DA, Bal T (1997) Sleep and arousal: thalamocortical mechanisms. *Annu Rev Neurosci*. **20**:185–215.

McHenry PL, Farris JV, Jordan JW, Morris SN (1977) Comparative study of cardiovascular function and premature ventricular complexes in smokers and non-smokers during maximal treadmill exercise. *Am J Cardiol*. **39**:493–498.

Mercadier JJ, Lompre AM, Duc P, Boheler KR, Fraysse JB, Wisnewsky C, et al (1990) Altered sarcoplasmatic reticulum Ca++-ATPase gene expression in the human ventricle. *J Clin Invest*. **85**:305-309.

Meredith IT, Broughton A, Jennings GL, Esler MD (1991) Evidence of a selective increase in cardiac sympathetic activity in patients with sustained ventricular arrhythmias. *N Engl J Med*. **325**:618–624.

MERIT-HF Study Group (1999) Effect of metoprolol CR/XL in chronic heart failure: Metoprolol CR/XL randomized intervention trial in congestive heart failure (MERIT-HF). *Lancet*. **353**:2001-2007.

Michaels DC, Matyas E, Jalife J (1987) Mechanism of sino atrial pacemaker synchronization: a new hypothesis. *Circ Res*. **61**:704–714.

Moncada S, Herman AG, Higgs EA, Vane JR (1977) Differential formation of prostacyclin (PGX or PGI2) by layers of arterial wall: an explanation for the anti-thrombotic properties of the vascular endothelium. *Thromb Res*. **11**:323–344.

Monnet X, Ghaleh B, Colin P, Parent-De-Curzon O, Giudicelli JF, Berdeaux A, Bize A (2001) Heart rate reduction by ivabradine exerts both preventive and curative effects on exercise-induced myocardial stunning in dogs. *Eur Heart J*. 22(Abstract S):P3697.

Monteggia LM, Eisch AJ, Tang MD, Kaczmarek LK, Nestler EJ (2000) Cloning and localization of the hyperpolarization-activated cyclic nucleotide-gated channel family in rat brain. *Mol Brain Res*. **81**:129–139.

Moosmang S, Biel M, Hofmann F, Ludwig A (1999) Differential distribution of four hyperpolarization-activated cation channels in mouse brain. *Biol Chem*. **380**:975–980.

Moosmang S, Stieber J, Zong X, Biel M, Hofmann F, Ludwig A (2001) Cellular expression and functional characterization of four hyperpolarization-activated pacemaker channels in cardiac and neuronal tissues. *Eur J Biochem*. **268**:1646–1652.

Moroni A, Barbuti A, Altomare C, Viscomi C, Morgan J, Baruscotti M, et al (2000) Kinetic and ionic properties of the human HCN2 pacemaker channel. *Pflügers Arch*. **439**:618–626.

Moroni A, Vaccari T, Bianchi ME, Beltrame M, DiFrancesco D (1999) Molecular characterization of the pacemaker channel of the heart: HCN members expressed in sinoatrial node. *Biophys J*. **76**:A210.

Mulieri LA, Hasenfuss G, Leavitt B, Allen PD, Alpert NR (1992) Altered myocardial force-frequency relation in human heart failure. *Circulation*. **85**:1743-1750.

Munsch T, Pape HC (1999) Modulation of the hyperpolarization-activated cation current of rat thalamic relay neurones by intracellular pH. *J Physiol*. **519**:493–504.

Murray PA, Vatner SF (1981) Reduction of maximal coronary vasodilator capacity in conscious dogs with severe right ventricular hypertrophy. *Circ Res*. **48**:25–33.

Musialek P, Lei M, Brown HF, Paterson DJ, Casadei B (1997) Nitric oxide can increase heart rate by stimulating the hyperpolarization-activated inward current, I_f. *Circ Res*. **81**:60–68.

Myers RW, Pearlman AS, Hyman RM, Goldstein RA, Kent KM, Goldstein RE, et al (1974) Beneficial effects of vagal stimulation and bradycardia during experimental acute myocardial ischemia. *Circulation.* **49**:943–947.

Nabauer M, Beuckelmann DJ, Erdmann E (1993) Characteristics of transient outward current in human ventricular myocytes from patients with terminal heart failure. *Circ Res.* **73**:386–394.

Neumann J, Schmitz W, Scholz H, von Meyerinck L, Doring V, Kalmar P (1988) Increase in myocardial Gi-proteins in heart failure. *Lancet.* **2**:936–937.

Noble D, Tsien RW (1968) The kinetics and rectifier properties of the slow potassium current in calf Purkinje fibres. *J Physiol.* **195**:185–214.

Nolan J, Batin PD, Andrews R, Lindsay SJ, Brooksby P, Mullen M, et al (1998) Prospective study of heart rate variability and mortality in chronic heart failure. *Circulation.* **98**:1510–1516.

Nolan J, Flapan AD, Capewell S, MacDonald TM, Neilson JM, Ewing DJ (1992) Decreased cardiac parasympathetic activity in chronic heart failure and its relation to left ventricular function. *Br Heart J.* **67**:482-486.

Norwegian Multi-center Study Group (1981) Timolol-induced reduction in mortality and reinfarction in patients surviving acute myocardial infarction. *N Engl J Med.* **304**:801–807.

Ong JC, Sarma JSM, Venkataraman K, Levin SR, Singh BN (1993) Circadian rhythmicity of heart rate and QTc interval in diabetic autonomic neuropathy. Implications for the mechanisms of sudden cardiac death. *Am Heart J.* **125**:744–752.

Opasich C, Rapezzi C, Lucci D, Gorini M, Pozzar F, Zanelli E, et al, on behalf of the Italian Network on Congestive Heart Failure (IN-CHF) Investigators (2001). Precipitating factors and decision-making processes of short-term worsening heart failure despite 'optimal treatment'. *Am J Cardiol.* **88**: 332-387.

Pachucki J, Burmeister LA, Larsen PR (1999) Thyroid hormone regulates hyperpolarization-activated cyclic nucleotide-gated channel (HCN2) mRNA in the rat heart. *Circ Res.* **85**:498–503.

Packer M (1998) β-adrenergic blockade in chronic heart failure: principles, progress, and practice. *Prog Cardiovasc Dis.* **41(Suppl 1)**:39–52.

Packer M, Carver JR, Rodeheffer RJ, Ivanhoe RJ, DiBianco R, Zeldis SM, et al (1991) Effect of oral milrinone on mortality in severe chronic heart failure. The PROMISE Study Research Group. *N Engl J Med.* **325**:1468–1475.

Packer M, Coats AJ, Fowler MB, Katus HA, Krum H, Mohacsi P, et al for The Carvedilol Prospective Randomized Cumulative Survival Study Group (2001) Effect of carvedilol on survival in severe chronic heart failure. *N Engl J Med.* **344**:1651–1658.

Palatini P, Julius S (1999) Relevance of heart rate as a risk factor in hypertension. *Curr Hypertens Rep.* **1**:219–224.

Palmer RMJ, Ferrige AG, Moncada S (1987) Nitric oxide release accounts for the biological activity of endothelium–derived relaxing factor. *Nature.* **327**:524–526.

Pape HC (1996) Queer current and pacemaker: the hyperpolarization-activated cation current in neurons. *Annu Rev Physiol.* **58**:299–327.

Pape HC, Mager R (1992) Nitric oxide controls oscillatory activity in thalamocortical neurons. *Neuron.* **9**:441–448.

Parker GW, Michael LH, Hartley CJ, Shinner JE, Entman ML (1990) Central β-adrenergic mechanisms may modulate ischemic ventricular fibrillation in pigs. *Circ Res.* **66**:259–270.

Patberg KW, Plotnikov A, Gainullin R, Quarmina A, Samaniengo L, Danilo P, et al (2001) Cardiac memory is associated with alterations in the cAMP responsive element binding protein and its phosphorylated form. *Pacing Clin Electrophysiol.* **24**:645.

Pepine CJ, Abrams J, Marks RG, Morris JJ, Scheidt SS, Handberg E (1994) Characteristics of a contemporary population with angina pectoris. TIDES Investigators. *Am J Cardiol.* **74**:226–231.

Perski A, Olsson G, Landou C, de Faire U, Theorell T, Hamsten A (1992) Minimum heart rate and coronary atherosclerosis: independent relations to global severity and rate of progression of angiographic lesions in men with myocardial infarction at a young age. *Am Heart J.* **123**:609–616.

Pfeifer A, Dostmann WRG, Sausbier M, Klatt P, Ruth P, Hofmann F (1999) cGMP-dependent protein kinases: structure and function. *Rev Physiol Biochem Pharmacol.* **135**:105–149.

Plotnikov A, Shvilkin A, deGroot J, Xiong W, Rosenshtraukh L, Feinmark S, et al (2001) Interactions between antiarrhythmic drugs and cardiac memory. *Cardiovasc Res.* **50**:335–344.

Pollare T, Lithell H, Selinus I, Berne C (1989) Sensitivity to insulin during treatment with atenolol and metoprolol: a randomised, double blind study of effects on carbohydrate and lipoprotein metabolism in hypertensive patients. *BMJ.* **298**:1152–1157.

Porciatti F, Pelzmann B, Cerbai E, Schaffer P, Pino R, Berhart E, et al (1997) The pacemaker current I_f in single human atrial myocytes and the effect of β-adrenoceptor and A_1-adenosine receptor stimulation. *Br J Pharmacol.* **122**:963–969.

Post SR, Hammond HK, Insel PA (1999) β-adrenergic receptors and receptor signaling in heart failure. *Annu Rev Pharmacol Toxicol.* **39**:343–360.

Pousset F, Copie X, Lechat P, Jaillon P, Boissel JP, Hetzel M, et al (1996) Effects of bisoprolol on heart rate variability in heart failure. *Am J Cardiol.* **77**:612–617.

Prinzen FW, Augustijn CH, Arts T, Allessie MA, Reneman RS (1990) Redistribution of myocardial fiber strain and blood flow by asynchronous activation. *Am J Physiol.* **259**:H300–H308.

Ragueneau I, Laveille C, Jochemsen R, Resplandy G, Funck-Bretano C, Jaillon P (1998) Pharmacokinetic-pharmacodynamic modelling of the effects of ivabradine, a direct sinus node inhibitor, on heart rate in healthy volunteers. *Clin Pharmacol Ther.* **64**:192-203.

Ramahi TM (2000) Beta blocker therapy for chronic heart failure. *Am Fam Physician.* **62**: 2267–2274.

Ramirez JM, Richter DW (1996) The neuronal mechanisms of respiratory rhythm generation. *Curr Opin Neurobiol.* **6**:817–825.

Reimer KA, Jennings RB (1979) The "wave-front" phenomenon of myocardial ischemic cell death: II Transmural progression of necrosis within the framework of ischemic bed size (myocardium at risk) and collateral flow. *Lab Invest.* **40**:633–644.

Reiter MJ (2000) Antiarrhythmic impact of anti-ischemic, anti-failure and other cardiovascular strategies. *Card Electrophysiol Rev.* **4**:194–205.

Reiter MJ, Reiffel JA (1998) Importance of β blockade in the therapy of serious ventricular arrhythmias. *Am J Cardiol.* **82**:(4A):9I.

Renaudon B, Bois P, Bescond J, Lenfant J (1997) Acetylcholine modulates I_f and $I_{K(Ach)}$ via different pathways in rabbit sino-atrial node cells. *J Mol Cell Cardiol.* **29**:969–975.

Renaudon B, Lenfant J, Decressac S, Bois P (2000) Thyroid hormone increases the conductance density of f-channels in rabbit sino-atrial node cells. *Receptors Channels.* **7**:1–8.

Reneland R, Alvarez E, Andersson PE, Haenni A, Byberg L, Lithell H (2000) Induction of insulin resistance by beta-blockade but not ACE-inhibition: long-term treatment with atenolol or trandolapril. *J Hum Hypertens.* **14**:175–180.

Ricard P, Danilo P Jr, Cohen IS, Burkhoff D, Rosen MR (1999) A role of the renin-angiotensin system in the evolution of cardiac memory. *J Cardiovasc Electrophysiol.* **10**:545–551.

Rich MW, Saini JS, Kleiger RE, Carney RM, Velde A, Freedland KE (1988) Correlation of heart rate variability with clinical and angiographic variables and late mortality after coronary angiography. *Am J Cardiol.* **69**:714–717.

Robinson RB, Yu H, Chang F, Cohen IS (1997) Developmental change in the voltage-dependence of the pacemaker current, I_f, in rat ventricle cells. *Pflügers Arch.* **433**:533–535.

Rosen MR (2001) The heart remembers: clinical implications. *Lancet.* **357**:468–471.

Rosen MR, Cohen IS, Danilo P Jr, Steinberg SF (1998) The heart remembers. *Cardiovasc Res.* **40**:469–482.

Rosenbaum MB, Blanco HH, Elizari MV, Lazzari JQ, Davidenko JM (1982) Electrotonic modulation of the T wave and cardiac memory. *Am J Cardiol.* **50**:213–222.

Rosenbaum MB, Blanco HH, Elizari MV, Lazzari JQ, Vetulli HM (1983) Electrotonic modulation of ventricular repolarization and cardiac memory. In: Rosenbaum MB, Elizari W, (eds.) *Frontiers of Cardiac Electrophysiology*. Boston, Mass: Martinus Nijhoff; 67–99.

Rossen JD, Oskarson H, Minor RL Jr, Talman CL, Winniford MD (1994) Effect of adenosine antagonism on metabolically mediated coronary vasodilation in humans. *Am J Cardiol.* **23**:1421–1426.

Ryu KH, Tanaka N, Ross J (1996) Effect of a sinus node inhibitor on the normal and failing rabbit heart. *Basic Res Cardiol.* **91**:131-139.

Sa Cunha R, Pannier B, Benetos A, Siche JP, London GM, Mallion JM, et al (1997) Association between high heart rate and high arterial rigidity in normotensive and hypertensive subjects. *J Hypertens.* **15(12 Pt 1)**:1423–1430.

Sadoshima JI, Izumo S (1993) Mechanical stretch activates multiple signal transduction pathways in cardiac myocytes: potential involvement of an autocrine/paracrine mechanism. *EMBO J.* **12**:1681–1692.

Sadoshima JI, Jahn L, Takahashi T, Kulik TJ, Izumo S (1992) Molecular characterization of the stretch-induced adaptation of cultured cardiac cells. *J Biol Chem.* **267**:10551–10560.

Sakmann B, Noma A, Trautwein W (1983) Acetylcholine activation of single muscarinic K^+ channels in isolated pacemaker cells of the mammalian heart. *Nature.* **303**:250–253.

Santoro B, Chen S, Lüthi A, Pavlidis P, Shumyatsky GP, Tibbs GR, et al (2000) Molecular and functional heterogeneity of hyperpolarization-activated pacemaker channels in the mouse CNS. *J Neurosci.* **20**:5264–5275.

Santoro B, Grant SGN, Bartsch D, Kandel ER (1997) Interactive cloning with the SH3 domain of N-src identifies a new brain specific ion channel protein, with homology to Eag and cyclic nucleotide-gated channels. *Proc Natl Acad Sci U S A.* **94**:14815–14820.

Santoro B, Liu DT, Yao H, Bartsch D, Kandel ER, Siegelbaum SA, et al (1998) Identification of a gene encoding a hyperpolarization-activated pacemaker channel of brain. *Cell.* **93**:717–729.

Santoro B, Tibbs GR (1999) The HCN gene family: molecular basis of the hyperpolarization-activated pacemaker channels. In: Molecular and functional diversity of ion channels and receptors. *Ann N Y Acad Sci.* **868**:741–764.

Sartiani L, Cerbai E, DePaoli P, Bizzarri F, DiCiolla F, Davoli G, et al (1999) β1, β2 and β3 Adrenoceptor subtypes differently modulate the pacemaker current in human ventricular myocytes. *Circulation.* **100(Suppl)**:I-488 (Abstract).

Satoh H, Sperelakis N (1993) Hyperpolarization-activated inward current in embryonic chick cardiac myocytes: developmental changes and modulation by isoproterenol and carbachol. *Eur J Pharmacol.* **240**:283–290.

Satoh TO, Yamada M (2000) A bradycardiac agent ZD7288 blocks the hyperpolarization-activated current $(I_{(h)})$ in retinal rod photoreceptors. *Neuropharmacology.* **39**:1284–1291.

Saul JP, Arai Y, Berger RD, Lilly LS, Colucci WS, Cohen RJ (1988) Assessment of autonomic regulation in chronic congestive heart failure by heart rate spectral analysis. *Am J Cardiol.* **61**:1292–1299.

Scamps F, Mayoux E, Charlemagne D, Vassort G (1990) Calcium current in single cells isolated from normal and hypertrophied rat heart. Effects of β-adrenergic stimulation. *Circ Res.* **67**:199–208.

Schaper W (1993) New paradigms for collateral vessel growth. *Basic Res Cardiol.* **88**:193–198.

Schwartz JS, Bache RJ (1985) Effect of arteriolar dilation on coronary artery diameter distal to coronary stenosis. *Am J Physiol.* **249 (5, part 2)**:H981–H988.

Schwartz PJ (1985) The idiopathic long QT interval syndrome: progress and questions. *Am Heart J.* **109**:399–405.

Seccareccia F, Pannozzo F, Dima F, Minoprio A, Menditto A, Lo Noce C, et al, Malattie Cardiovascolari Aterosclerotiche Istituto Superiore di Sanita Project (2001) Heart rate as a predictor of mortality: the MATISS project. *Am J Public Health.* **91**:1258–1263.

Seifert R, Scholten A, Gauss R, Mincheva A, Lichter P, Kaupp UB (1999) Molecular characterization of a slowly gating human hyperpolarization-activated channel predominantly expressed in thalamus, heart, and testis. *Proc Natl Acad Sci U S A.* **96**:9391–9396.

Shah PK (1997) Pathophysiology of acute coronary syndromes. *Am J Cardiol.* **79**:790–792.

Shah PK (1998) Role of inflammation and metalloproteinases in plaque disruption and thrombosis. *Vasc Med.* **3**:199–206.

Shaper AG, Wannamethee G, Macfarlane PW, Walker M (1993) Heart rate, ischaemic heart disease, and sudden cardiac death in middle-aged British men. *Br Heart J.* **70**:49–55.

Sherman CT, Litvack F, Grundfest W, Lee M, Hickey A, Chaux A, et al (1986) Coronary angioscopy in patients with unstable angina pectoris. *N Engl J Med.* **315**:913–919.

Shi W, Wymore R, Yu H, Wu J, Wymore RT, Pan Z, et al (1999) Distribution and prevalence of hyperpolarization-activated cation channel (HCN) mRNA expression in cardiac tissues. *Circ Res.* **85**:e1–e6.

Shimoni Y, Fiset C, Clark RB, Dixon JE, McKinnon D, Giles WR (1997) Thyroid hormone regulates postnatal expression of transient K$^+$ channel isoforms in rat ventricle. *J Physiol (Lond.).* **500**:65–73.

Shinbane JS, Wood MA, Jensen DN, Ellenbogen KA, Fitzpatrick AP, Scheinman MM (1997) Tachycardia-induced cardiomyopathy: a review of animal models and clinical studies. *J Am Coll Cardiol.* **29**:709–715.

Shinke T, Takeuchi M, Takaoka H, Yokoyama M (1999) Beneficial effects of heart rate reduction on cardiac mechanics and energetics in patients with left ventricular dysfunction. *Jpn Circ J.* **63**:957–964.

Shvilkin A, Danilo P Jr, Wang J, Burkhoff D, Anyukhovsky EP, Sosunov EA, et al (1998) Evolution and resolution of long-term cardiac memory. *Circulation.* **97**:1810–1817.

Simon L, Ghaleh B, Puybasset L, Giudicelli J-F, Berdeaux A (1995) Coronary and hemodynamic effects of S 16257, a new bradycardic agent, in resting and exercising conscious dogs. *J Pharmacol Exp Ther.* **275**:659–666.

Singer W, Gray CM (1995) Visual feature integration and the temporal correlation hypothesis. *Annu Rev Neurosci.* **18**:555–586.

Singh BN (1990) Advantages of β-blockers versus antiarrhythmic agents and calcium antagonists in secondary prevention of myocardial infarction. *Am J Cardiol.* **66**:9C–20C.

Singh BN (1998) Antiarrhythmic drugs: A re-orientation in light of recent developments in the control of disorders of cardiac rhythm. *Am J Cardiol.* **81**:3D–13D.

Singh BN (1999) The relevance of sympathetic activity in the pharmacological treatment of chronic stable angina. *Can J Cardiol.* **15(Suppl A)**: 15A–121A.

Singh BN, Vanhoutte PM (2002). *Selective and specific I_f current inhibition in cardiovascular disease.* London, UK: Lippincott Williams & Wilkins; p 1.

Skantze HB, Kaplan J, Pettersson K, Manuck S, Blomqvist N, Kyes R, et al (1998) Psychosocial stress causes endothelial injury in cynomolgus monkeys via B1-adrenoceptor activation. *Atherosclerosis.* **136**:153–161.

Skarfors ET, Lithell HO, Selinus I, Aberg H (1989) Do antihypertensive drugs precipitate diabetes in predisposed men? *BMJ.* **298**:1147–1152.

Smith PL, Baukrowitz TM, Yellen G (1996) The inward rectification mechanism of the HERG cardiac potassium channel. *Nature.* **379**:833–836.

Steenbergen C, Hill ML, Jennings RB (1985) Volume regulation and plasma membrane injury in aerobic, anaerobic, and ischemic myocardium in vitro. *Circ Res.* **57**:864–875.

Steinbeck G, Andersen D, Bach P, Haberi R, Oleff M, Hoffman E, et al (1992) A comparison of electrophysiologically guided antiarrhythmic drug therapy with β-blocker therapy to patients with symptomatic sustained tachyarrhythmias. *N Engl J Med.* **327**:987–993.

Stokes J III, Kannel WB, Wolf PA, Cupples A, D'Agostino RB (1987) The relative importance of selected factors for various manifestations of cardiovascular disease among men and women from 35–64 years old: 30 years of follow–up in the Framingham Study. *Circulation.* **75(Suppl V)**:V–65–73.

Strawn WB, Bondjers G, Kaplan JR, Manuck SB, Schwenke DC, Hansson GK, et al (1991) Endothelial dysfunction in response to psychosocial stress in monkeys. *Circ Res.* **68**:1270–1279.

Sun Z-Q, Ojamaa K, Coetzee WA, Artman M, Klein I (2000) Effects of thyroid hormone on action potential and repolarizing currents in rat ventricular myocytes. *Am J Physiol.* **278**:E302–E307.

Swynghedauw B (1999) Molecular mechanisms of myocardial remodeling. *Physiol Rev.* **79**:215–262.

Tan HL, Hou CJ, Lauer MR, Sung RJ (1995) Electrophysiologic mechanisms of the long QT interval syndromes and torsades de pointes. *Ann Intern Med.* **122**(9):701–714.

Tattersfield AE (1991) Respiratory function in the elderly and the effects of beta blockade. *Cardiovasc Drugs Ther.* **4(Suppl 6)**:1229–1232.

Thaulow E, Erikssen J (1991) How important is heart rate? *J Hypertens.* **9**:S27–S30.

The β-blocker Evaluation of Survival Trial Investigators (2001) A trial of the β-blocker bucindolol in patients with advanced chronic heart failure. *N Engl J Med.* **344**:1659–1667.

Thollon C, Bodouard JP, Cambarrat C, Lesage L, Reure H, Delescluse I, et al (1997) Stereospecific in vitro and in vivo effects of the new sinus node inhibitor (+)-S16257. *Eur J Pharmacol.* **339**:43-51.

Thollon C, Cambarrat C, Vian J, Prost JF, Peglion JL, Vilaine JP (1994) Electrophysiological effects of S 16257, a novel sino-atrial node modulator, on rabbit and guinea-pig cardiac preparations: comparison with UL-FS 49. *Br J Pharmacol.* **112**:37–42.

Thuringer D, Lauribe P, Escande D (1992) A hyperpolarization-activated inward current in human myocardial cells. *J Mol Cell Cardiol.* **24**:451–455.

Tomaselli G, Marban E (1999) Electrophysiological remodeling in hypertrophy and heart failure. *Cardiovasc Res.* **42**:270–283.

Tomaselli GF, Beuckelmann DJ, Calkins HG, Berger RD, Kessler PD, Lawrence JH, et al (1994) Sudden cardiac death in heart failure. The role of abnormal repolarization. *Circulation.* **90**:2534–2539.

Treasure CB, Klein JL, Weintraub WS, Talley JD, Stillabower ME, Kosinski AS, et al (1995) Beneficial effects of cholesterol-lowering therapy on the coronary endothelium in patients with coronary artery disease. *N Engl J Med.* **332**:491–497.

Tsuji H, Venditi LJ, Manders ES (1994) Reduced heart rate variability and mortality risk in an elderly cohort. The Framingham heart study. *Circulation.* **90**:878–883.

Tuininga YS, van Veldhuisen DJ, Brouwer J, Haaksma J, Crijns HJ, Man in 't Veld AJ, et al (1994) Heart rate variability in left ventricular dysfunction and heart failure: effects and implications of drug treatment. *Br Heart J.* **72**:509-513.

Ulens C, Tytgat J (2001) Functional heteromerization of HCN1 and HCN2 pacemaker channels. *J Biol Chem.* **276**:6069–6072.

Ungerer M, Bohm M, Elce JS, Erdmann E, Lohse MJ (1993) Altered expression of β-adrenergic receptor kinase and β 1-adrenergic receptors in the failing human heart. *Circulation.* **87**:454–463.

Vaca L, Stieber J, Zong X, Ludwig A, Hofmann F, Biel M (2000) Mutations in the S4 domain of a pacemaker channel alter its voltage dependence. *FEBS Lett.* **479**:35–40.

Vaccari T, Moroni A, Rocchi M, Gorza L, Bianchi ME, Beltrame M, et al D (1999) The human gene for HCN2, a pacemaker channel of the heart. *Biochim Biophys Acta.* **1446**:419–425.

Valenzuela C, Delpon E, Franqueza L, Gay P, Perez O, Tamargo J, et al (1996) Class III antiarrhythmic effects of zatebradine. Time, state-, use-, and voltage-dependent block of hKv 1.5 channels. *Circulation.* **94**:562-570.

Van Bogaert P, Goethals M (1987) Pharmacological influence of specific bradycardic agents on the pacemaker current of sheep cardiac Purkinje fibres. A comparison between three different molecules. *Eur Heart J.* **8(Suppl L)**:35–42.

Van Camp JR, Brunsting LA 3rd, Childs KF, Bolling SF (1995) Functional recovery after ischemia: warm versus cold cardioplegia. *Ann Thorac Surg.* **59**:795–802; discussion 802–803.

Varnum MD, Black KD, Zagotta WN (1995) Molecular mechanism for ligand discrimination of cyclic nucleotide-gated channels. *Neuron.* **15**:619–625.

Vatner SF, Baig H (1979) Importance of heart rate in determining the effects of sympathomimetic amines on regional myocardial function and blood flow in conscious dogs with acute myocardial ischemia. *Circ Res.* **45**:793–803.

Vatner SF, Higgins CB, Franklin D, Braunwald E (1972) Role of tachycardia in mediating the coronary hemodynamic response to severe exercise. *J Appl Physiol.* **32**:380–385.

Vita JA, Treasure CB, Nabel EG, McLenachan JM, Fish RD, Yeung AC, et al (1990) Coronary vasomotor response to acetylcholine relates to risk factors for coronary artery disease. *Circulation.* **81**:491–497.

Waagstein F, Bristow MR, Swedberg K, Camerini F, Fowler MB, Silver MA, et al for the metoprolol in dilated cardiomyopathy (MDC) trial study group (1993) Beneficial effects of metoprolol in idiopathic dilated cardiomyopathy. *Lancet.* **342**:1441-1446.

Walsh RW, Porter CB, Starling MR, O'Rourke MA (1984) Beneficial hemodynamic effects of intravenous and oral diltiazem in severe congestive heart failure. *J Am Coll Cardiol.* **3**:1044-1050.

Warmke JW, Ganetzky B (1994) A family of potassium channel genes related to *eag* in *Drosophila* and mammals. *Proc Natl Acad Sci U S A.* **91**:3438–3442.

White S, Patrick T, Higgins CB, Vatner SF, Franklin D, Braunwald E (1971) Effects of altering ventricular rate on blood flow distribution in conscious dogs. *Am J Physiol.* **221**:1402–1407.

Wiesfeld AC, Crijns HJ, Tuininga YS, Lie KI (1996) β-adrenergic blockade in the treatment of sustained ventricular tachycardia or ventricular fibrillation. *Pacing Clin Electrophysiol.* **19**:1026–1035.

Wilhelmsen L, Berglund G, Elmfeldt D, Elmfeldt D, Tibblin G, Wedel H, et al (1986) The multifactor primary prevention trial in Göteborg, Sweden. *Eur Heart J.* **7**:279–288.

Wilson FN, MacLeod AG, Barker PS, Johnston FD (1934) The determination and the significance of the areas of the ventricular deflections of the electrocardiogram. *Am Heart J.* **10**:46–61.

Wit AL, Rosen MR (1986) Afterdepolarizations and triggered activity. In: Fozzard H, (ed.) *The Heart and Cardiovascular System.* New York, NY: Raven Press; 1449–1490.

Wollmuth LP, Hille B (1992) Ionic selectivity of I_h channels of rod photoreceptors in tiger salamanders. *J Gen Physiol.* **100**:749–765.
Woo MA, Stevenson WG, Moser DK, Middlekauff HR (1994) Complex heart rate variability and serum norepinephrine levels in patients with advanced heart failure. *J Am Coll Cardiol.* **23**:565–569.
Woo MA, Stevenson WG, Moser DK, Trelease RB, Harper RM (1992) Patterns of beat to beat heart rate variability in advanced heart failure. *Am Heart J.* **123**:704–710.
Xiao RP, Ji X, Lakatta EG (1995) Functional coupling of the β2-adrenoceptor to a pertussis toxin-sensitive G protein in cardiac myocytes. *Mol Pharmacol.* **47**:322–329.
Yamabe H, Okumura K, Ishizaka H, Tsuchiya T, Yasue H (1992) Role of endothelium-derived nitric oxide in myocardial reactive hyperemia. *Am J Physiol.* **263(1, part 2)**:H8–H14.
Yamanishi K, Fujita M, Sasayama S, Nakajima H, Asanoi H, Ohno A (1988) Functional characteristics of nonischemic regions during pacing induced myocardial ischemia in angina pectoris. *Am J Cardiol.* **61**:1214–1218.
Yanagisawa M, Kurihara H, Kimura S, Tomabe Y, Kohayashi M, Mitsui Y, et al (1988) A novel potent vasoconstrictor peptide produced by vascular endothelial cells. *Nature.* **332**:411–415.
Yasui K, Liu W, Opthof T, Kada K, Lee JK, Kamiya K, et al (2001) I_f current and spontaneous activity in mouse embryonic ventricular myocytes. *Circ Res.* **88**:536–542.
Yatani A, Okabe K, Codina J, Birnbaumer L, Brown AM (1990) Heart rate regulation by G proteins acting on the cardiac pacemaker channel. *Science.* **249**:1163–1166.
Yeung AC, Vekshtein VI, Krantz DS, Vita JA, Ryan TJ Jr, Ganz P, et al (1991) The effect of atherosclerosis on the vasomotor response of coronary arteries to mental stress. *N Engl J Med.* **325**:1551–1556.
Yoo S, Lee SH, Choi BH, Yeom JB, Ho WK, Earm YE (1998) Dual effect of nitric oxide on the hyperpolarization-activated inward current (I_f) in sino-atrial node cells of the rabbit. *J Mol Cell Cardiol.* **30**:2729–2738.
Yu H, Chang F, Cohen IS (1993) Pacemaker current exists in ventricular myocytes. *Circ Res.* **72**:232–236.
Yu H, Chang F, Cohen IS (1995) Pacemaker current I_f in adult canine cardiac ventricular myocytes. *J Physiol.* **485**:469–483.
Yu H, Gao J, Wang H, Wymore R, Steinberg S, McKinnon D, et al (2000) Effects of the renin-angiotensin system on the current I_{to} in epicardial and endocardial ventricular myocytes from the canine heart. *Circ Res.* **86**:1062–1068.
Yu H, McKinnon D, Dixon JE, Gao J, Wymore R, Cohen IS, et al (1999) Transient outward current, I_{to1}, is altered in cardiac memory. *Circulation.* **99**:1898–1905.
Yusuf S, Peto R, Lewis J, Sleight P (1985) β-blockade during myocardial infarction: an overview of randomized trials. *Prog Cardiovasc Dis.* **27**:335–355.
Zagotta WN, Siegelbaum SA (1996) Structure and function of cyclic nucleotide-gated channels. *Annu Rev Neurosci.* **19**:235–263.
Zaza A, Rocchetti M, DiFrancesco D (1996) Modulation of the hyperpolarization-activated current (I_f) by adenosine in rabbit sinoatrial myocytes. *Circulation.* **94**:734–741.
Zei PC, Aldrich R (1998) Voltage-dependent gating of single wild-type and S4 mutant KAT1 inward rectifier potassium channels. *J Gen Physiol.* **112**:679–713.
Zong X, Stieber J, Ludwig A, Hofmann F, Biel M (2001) A single histidine residue determines the pH sensitivity of the pacemaker channel HCN2. *J Biol Chem.* **276**:6313–6319.
Zong X, Zucker H, Hofmann F, Biel M (1998) Three amino acids in the C-linker are major determinants of gating in cyclic nucleotide-gated channels. *EMBO J.* **17**:353–362.
Zuanetti G, Neilson JMM, Latini R, Santoro E, Maggioni AP, Ewing DJ (1996) Prognostic significance of heart rate variability in post myocardial infarction patients in the fibrinolytic era. The GISSI-II results. *Circulation.* **94**:432–436.

SUBJECT INDEX

Accumulation 38
Acebutolol 103
Acetylcholine
    I_f current regulation 11–12
        activation shift 5–6, 34
    parasympathetic effects 5
Action potentials
    duration, heart failure 19, 25–26
    I_f current see I_f current
    phases 3, 89, 90
    sinus node 62
Activation pathways 37–44
    alteration, causes 37, 44
    atrial pacing experiments 41–43
        atrial gradient calculation 41–42
        left vs right pacing 42–43
        methods 38, 43
        Ta waves 41–43
    ventricular pacing experiments 38–41
        angiotensin II role 40
        methods 37–38
        QRS complexes 38, 39
        T wave alteration 38–41
    see also pacemaker activity
Actomyosin system 85
Adenosine, pacemaker regulation 12, 14
Adrenergic receptors
    α-receptors 24
    adenosine release 12
    β-receptors
        antagonists see β-blockers
        subtypes 24–25
    heart rate acceleration 4, 5
    modulation 22, 24–25
        β-adrenoceptor kinase (βARK) 24
        G proteins 24–25
Adventitia remodeling 69
Age, cardiovascular morbidity/mortality 96, 97, 100, 104, 105
Alinidine 7
Angina
    exercise tolerance test (ETT) 77, 80
    stable
        β-blocker efficacy 81–83, 84
        heart rate 77
        ischemic preconditioning 74
        ivabradine efficacy 77–84
        symptoms 77
    unstable 72–73
Angiotensin II
    cardiac memory role 40, 44
    hypertrophic gene re-expression 22

Arrhythmias 19
    activation pathways 37, 44
    lethal ventricular 59
    see also activation pathways; pacemaker activity
Atherogenic diets 45
Atherosclerosis 69
    behavioral exacerbation 47–48
        β-blocker effects 48–50
    consequences
        ischemia 69
        thrombosis 72–73, 75
        see also coronary artery disease; myocardial ischemia
    epidemiology 45
    heart rate relationship
        clinical studies 45
        primate studies 45–51, 59
    plaques see atherosclerotic plaques
    progression 45
    psychosocial stress 47–48
    risk factors 46, 87
Atherosclerotic plaques 69, 75
    disruption/thrombosis 72–73, 75
Atrial gradient calculation 41–42
Atrial myocytes
    action potential phases 89, 90
    HCN channel expression 10
    I_f currents 14
Atrial pacing 38, 43
    left vs right pacing 42–43
    Ta waves 41–43
Autonomic nervous system
    heart rate and 87–89
    I_f current regulation 5–6, 11–12
    parasympathetic 5, 17, 87
    posture effect 89
    signaling pathways 17
    sinoatrial node innervation 5–6
    stretch receptors 88
    sympathetic see sympathetic nervous system

β-adrenoceptor kinase (βARK) 24
BAY y 5959, oxygen consumption effects 57
Behavior, atherogenic 47–48
β-adrenergic antagonists see β-blockers
β-blockers
    adverse effects 16, 82
    $β_1$- and $β_2$-selective agents 91
    $β_1$-selective agents 90–91
    bradycardia induction 1, 5, 68
        angina management 81–83
        atherogenesis effects 48–50
        clinical trials 101–103, 104
        endothelial injury reduction 50–51

Subject index

heart failure 90–91, 93, 101, 102
  myocardial infarction 101
clinical benefits 90, 95
contraindications 82–83
heart rate variability and 67–68
heterogeneity 90
ivabradine *versus* 81–83, 84
paradoxical vasoconstriction 82
see also specific drugs
Bisoprolol 91, 102, 103, 104
heart rate variability study 67–68
specificity 90–91
Bodwitch effect 86
Bradycardia 61–68
atherogenesis effects 45–52
mechanisms 61–63
pathological 61
pharmacological
  β-blocker-induced *see* β-blockers
  calcium channel blockers 16, 91
  SBAs 7–8, 16–17, 84, 91–93, 95
  see also heart rate reduction; *specific drugs*
sinus node ablation 45–47
Bucindolol 104

Calcium
channel blockers, heart rate reduction 16, 91
HCN channel modulation 34
heart rate and 16, 91
homeostasis alteration 87
myocardial contraction 85
Calcium channel blockers, heart rate reduction 16, 91
cAMP *see* cyclic AMP
Cardiac activation *see* activation pathways
Cardiac death, sudden *see* sudden cardiac death
Cardiac failure *see* heart rate
Cardiac glycosides, heart rate reduction 89
Cardiac Insufficiency BIsoprolol Studies (CIBIS I & II) 67–68, 91, 102
Cardiac ion channels
age-dependent expression 23
HCN channels *see* HCN channels
potassium channels 30, 33–34
Cardiac memory 37
angiotensin II role 40, 44
definition 38
quantification 38
ventricular pacing 38, 39
Cardiac muscle
contraction 85
electrophysiology 25–26
I_f current regulation 11–18
innervation *see* autonomic nervous system
stretch receptors 88

see also atrial myocytes; ventricular myocytes
Cardiac output, myocardial function 85
Cardiac repolarization, modification 37–45
Cardiomyopathy, electrophysiology 25–26
Cardiopulmonary stretch receptors 88
Cardiovascular disease
    epidemiology see epidemiological studies
    heart rate and 1, 61
    I_f current inhibition 1
    morbidity/mortality 61, 95–106
        age/gender 96, 97, 100, 104, 105
        elderly 99–100
        ethnicity 98, 105
        hypertension 99–100
        post-infarction 99, 100
        relative risk 97
        see also sudden cardiac death
    thyroid dysfunction 14–15
    see also heart rate; heart rate reduction; *specific conditions*
Cardiovascular Occupational Risk Factor Determination in Israel (CORDIS) study 95, 98
Carotid bifurcation atherosclerosis 47
Carvedilol 91, 103, 104
Cesium ions, HCN channel blockade 7, 33
cGMP see cyclic GMP
Chicago Employee Studies 95, 98, 104
Chronotropism 61
    acetylcholine effects 5–6
CIBIS I & II 67–68, 91, 102
Cold cardioplegia, ischemia reduction 56
Collateral blood flow 74–75
Congenital long QT syndrome 102
Congestive heart failure see heart failure
Cooling
    ischemia reduction 56
    pacemaker shifts 62–63
CORDIS study 95, 98
Coronary artery
    atherosclerosis see atherosclerosis
    blood flow see coronary blood flow
    circumflex 53, 54
    collaterals, protective role 74–75
    stenosis
        fixed and dynamic 70–72
        ST elevation 56
        see also coronary artery disease
Coronary artery disease
    angina see angina
    collaterals, protective effects 74–75
    heart rate
        atherogenesis and 45–51
        regulation in 55–59
        variability 65
        see also heart rate; heart rate reduction

inflammation 73
ischemic *see* myocardial ischemia
plaque disruption/thrombosis 72–73, 75
stable 70–72
unstable (acute syndromes) 72–75
    see also myocardial infarction
see also atherosclerosis; coronary artery
Coronary blood flow 1, 53
    autoregulation 70, 71
    cessation, consequences 73–74
        see also myocardial ischemia
    circumflex 53, 54
    collaterals 74–75
    exercise effects 53, 54, 55
    fixed and dynamic stenosis 70–72
    heart rate effects 58–59
    supply–demand 69–70
Coronary collaterals, protective role 74–75
Coronary reserve 55
Coronary steal, isoproterenol 58
Coronary thrombosis 72–73, 75
    see also atherosclerosis
Cyclic AMP
    calcium influx 87
    HCN activation 30, 32–33, 34
        direct binding *vs* PKA activation 12
        isoform variation 32–33
    I_f current regulation 5, 7, 10, 11–12, 17
Cyclic GMP
    HCN channels
        activation 32
        modulation 34
    nitric oxide and 14, 17
Cyclic nucleotide binding domain (CNBG) 30

Development
    I_f currents/channels 4–5, 21–22, 23, 26
    pathology *versus* 21–22, 23
Dilated cardiomyopathy (DCM)
    force–frequency relation 86–87
    heart rate influence 88
Dobutamine, oxygen consumption effects 57, 58
Dopamine, oxygen consumption effects 58

Elderly patients, cardiovascular disease 99–100
Endo-epi steal 71
Endothelium
    dysfunction and heart rate 50–51
    vascular tone modulation 71
Epidemiological studies 1, 59, 95
    atherogenesis 45
    cardiovascular mortality 95–98
    see also individual studies

Ethnicity, cardiovascular disease 98
Exercise
    collateral development 75
    heart rate and blood flow 53, 54, 55
    tolerance tests, angina 77, 80, 81

Force–frequency relation 86
    dilated cardiomyopathy vs control 86–87
    heart failure 86–87, 92
Framingham Heart study 1, 95–97, 104
    age/gender 96, 97, 100
    hypertension 99, 100
    sudden death 96
Frank-Starling's law 85

Gender, cardiovascular disease 96, 97, 100
Gene expression
    HCN channels 32, 35–36
        cardiac 9, 10, 35
        neuronal 10, 29, 35–36
        overexpression 14–15, 18
    myocardial hypertrophy 19
    myocardial ischemia 58
    pathology *versus* developmental 21–22, 23
    repolarization-induced 40
GISSI II trial 65
Glycosides, heart rate reduction 89
Goteborg Primary Prevention Trial 95, 98, 99
G proteins
    adrenergic receptor regulation 24–25
    I_f current regulation 11–12, 17
Growth factors, collateral development 75
Gruppo Italiano per lo Studio della Sopravvivenza nell'Infarto miocardico II (GISSI II trial) 65

HCN channels 29–36
    activation 30–33
        isoform variations 32–33
        time-course 30
        voltage-dependence 7, 30, 33
        see also cyclic AMP
    cesium ion blockade 7, 33
    cloning 8–9, 10, 29–30
    developmental expression 5, 21–22, 23
    electrophysiological properties 8–9
    functional properties 32
    gating models 30
    ionic permeability 5, 29, 33–34
    isoforms 3, 8–9, 29
        functional variation 32–33
        tissue variation 35–36
    modulation 34–35
        adrenergic 24
        see also I_f current, regulation

Subject index

overexpression 23
    hypertensive rats 20
    thyrotoxicosis 14–15, 18
sequence homologies 30, 33–34
single channel recording 7
structure/topology 9, 30, 31
tissue distribution 32, 35–36
    cardiac 9, 10, 35
    neuronal 10, 29, 35–36

Heart
    contraction 85
        activation pathways 37–44
        rate *see* heart rate
    development 4–5
        pathology *versus* 21–22, 23
    disease *see* cardiovascular disease
    evolution 37
    failure *see* heart failure
    oxygen consumption *see* myocardial oxygen consumption (MVO_2)
    pacemaker activity *see* pacemaker activity
    see also entries beginning cardiac

Heart failure
    autonomic dysfunction 87–89
        HRV and 88–89
        posture effect 89
    β-adrenergic dysfunction 22, 24–25
    electrophysiology 25–26
    force–frequency relation 86–87, 92
    gene expression in 19
    heart rate reduction in 56–58, 85–93, 103
        β-blockers 90–91, 93, 101, 102
        calcium blockers 91
        glycosides 89
        sinus node modulators 91–93
        see also heart rate reduction
    heart rate variability 65–67
    myocardial function 86–87
    prognosis 19
    tachycardia 93
        chronic, as cause 56
        compensatory 85

Heart rate 1, 61–68, 95–105
    acetylcholine effects 5–6
    angina 77
    atherogenesis relationship 45–51, 59
        clinical studies 45
        human males 46
        nonhuman primates 45–51, 59
        see also atherosclerosis
    autonomic control 5, 87–89
        see also autonomic nervous system
    coronary artery disease 45

decreased *see* bradycardia
endothelial dysfunction 50–51
exercise effects 53, 54, 55
gene expression effects 58
hypertension 99
increased *see* tachycardia
isoprenaline effects 6
modulation 5–6
mortality/morbidity relationship 61, 95–98, 103–104
    noncardiovascular 104–105
myocardial contraction relationship 86–87
myocardial function 85
myocardial infarction prognosis 59, 99, 100, 101
myocardial ischemia 53–60
oxygen consumption and 1, 56–58
'reactivity' 51
    see also psychosocial stress
reduction *see* heart rate reduction
regulation
    ischemia 55–59
    physiological 53–55
repolarization alteration 37–45
serum lipid effects 46
sympathomimetic response 56–58, 59
vascular effects 58–59
see also pacemaker activity

Heart rate reduction 1
    clinical implications 103, 105
    epidemiological data 1
    heart failure treatment 85–93, 101, 102, 103
    heart rate variability and 67–68
    morbidity/mortality effects 61, 95–105
    pharmacological 15–17, 85–86, 89–91
        adverse effects 16
        β-blockers *see* β-blockers
        calcium channel blockers 16, 91
        glycosides 89
        ivabradine efficacy 78, 92, 93
        potassium channels blockers 91
        specific bradycardic agents 7–8, 16–17, 84, 91–92
        see also specific drugs
    see also bradycardia

Heart rate variability (HRV) 61–68
    clinical implications 65–67
        coronary artery disease 65
        heart failure 65–67
        prognostic indicator 61, 63
    frequency domain 64, 66
    heart rate reduction and 67–68
    ivabradine effect 92
    measurement methods 61, 63–65
    nonlinear analysis 64–65

Subject index

RR intervals 64, 65
sympathovagal balance 88–89
time domain 64, 66, 89
Holter recordings 63, 65, 68
Hyperpolarization-activated cyclic nucleotide-gated channels *see* HCN channels
Hypertension and cardiovascular disease 19–21, 99–100
Hypertensive rats (SHR), ventricular myocyte currents 19–21
Hyperthyroidism, cardiac manifestations 14, 15, 18

I_f channels *see* HCN channels
I_f current 3–10
    activation 30–33
        curve 4, 5
        threshold changes 37
    atrial myocytes 14
    developmental patterns 4–5, 21
        pathological *versus* 21–22, 23
    experimental evidence for 4–5
    inhibition 7–8
        nonspecific 5, 92
        specific *see* specific bradycardic agents (SBA)
        see also β-blockers
    ion channel *see* HCN channels
    pacemaker depolarization 89
    properties 3–5
    regulation 5–6, 11–18, 29
        adenosine 12, 14
        autonomic 5–6, 11–12
        calcium 34
        cAMP 4, 5, 7, 10, 11–12, 30, 32, 34
        G proteins 11–12
        neurotransmitters 5–6, 11, 34
        nitric oxide 14, 34
        peptides 12, 13
        pH 34–35
        PKA activation 12, 34
        thyroid hormones 14–15
    safety mechanism 9, 10
    signaling pathways 12, 14–15, 17–18
    therapeutic target 15–17
    time-constant 5
    ventricular myocytes 19–28
I_h currents 10, 29
Industry, heart rate and mortality 95, 98
Inflammation, acute coronary syndromes 73
Intracellular calcium
    HCN channel modulation 34
    homeostasis 87
Intracellular pH, HCN channel modulation 34–35
Ischemia *see* myocardial ischemia
Ischemic necrosis 73–74
Ischemic preconditioning 74

Isoprenaline, heart rate effects 6
Isoproterenol, oxygen consumption effects 58
I_{to} currents
    developmental expression 21–22, 23
    repolarization phenomena 40–41, 44
Ivabradine 7, 91, 92, 93
    β-blockers *versus* 81–83
        propranolol *versus* 84
    heart rate reduction 7, 16, 78, 80, 83, 92, 93
        dose–response 79
    safety and tolerability 78, 80, 84
    stable angina trials 77–84
        attack frequency 79
        design 77–78
        efficacy 78–79
        results 78–81
        statistics 78
        time to ST depression 73, 77, 78–79, 81, 82
        withdrawal 79, 83
    use-dependent I_f block 16
    zatebradine *versus* 16–17

Luminal stenosis 69, 71
    see also atherosclerosis

Matrix metalloproteinases (MMPs), plaque disruption 72–73
Membrane capacitance, heart failure 25, 26–27
MERIT-HF Study Group 91, 102, 103
Metoprolol
    clinical trials 102, 103, 104
    endothelial injury 50
    specificity 90–91
Microvascular vasodilation 70, 75
Multicenter Post Infarction Program (MPIP) 65
Muscarinic receptors, parasympathetic effects 5
Myocardial contraction 85
    activation *see* activation pathways
    heart rate relationship 86–87
Myocardial function 85
Myocardial hibernation 74, 75
Myocardial hypertrophy
    gene expression 19
        developmental phenotype 21–22
    I_f current in hypertensive rats 19–21
    myocyte phenotypic change 19
    progression to heart failure 19
Myocardial infarction
    β-blocker trials 101–103
    heart rate and prognosis 59, 99, 100, 101
    necrosis prevention 74
    post-infarction mortality 99, 101
    thrombi formation 72–73

Subject index

Myocardial ischemia
    cold cardioplegia 56
    coronary collaterals, protective role 74–75
    definition 69
    ECG-ST segment elevation 55, 56
    gene expression 58
    heart rate
        reduction 15–17
        regulation 55–59
        sympathomimetics and 56–58, 59
    necrotic 73–74
    pathophysiology 69–75
        biochemical changes 70
        clinical implications 75
        fixed and dynamic stenosis 70–72
        inflammation 73
        plaque disruption 72–73
        supply–demand imbalance 69–70
        thrombosis 72–73, 75
        unstable (acute) syndromes 72–75
        vascular tone 70–72
        see also atherosclerosis
    preconditioning 74
    silent 69
    see also coronary blood flow
Myocardial oxygen consumption (MVO_2) 1, 53, 59–60
    insufficient *see* myocardial ischemia
    sympathomimetic effects 56–58
Myocardial stunning 74
Myocardium, heart rate effects 58–59

National Health and Nutrition Examination Survey *see* NHANES I
Nervous system
    autonomic *see* autonomic nervous system
    HCN channel expression 9, 10, 35–36
    pacemaker activity 29
        I_f-like currents (I_h) 10, 29
Neuropeptide Y (NPY), pacemaker regulation 12
Neurotransmitters, pacemaker regulation 11–12
NHANES I
    Epidemiological Follow-up Study (NNHEFS) 95, 97–98, 104
    heart rate and cardiovascular disease 95
Nitric oxide (NO)
    I_f current regulation 18, 34
        cGMP-mediated 14, 17
    vasodilation 72
Nitric oxide synthase (NOS) 72
Nonhuman primates, atherogenesis 45–51, 59

Oxprenolol 104
Oxygen consumption *see* myocardial oxygen consumption (MVO_2)

Pacemaker activity 3
    cardiac 3
    I_f current see I_f current
    neuronal 29
    phases 3, 89, 90
    repolarization and 37–44
    sites of 37
        sinoatrial see sinoatrial node
    synchronization 62–63
    see also activation pathways; heart rate
Pacemaker current see I_f current
Pacemaker shifts 62–63
Parasympathetic nervous system 5
    signaling 17
    sympathetic imbalance 87
P cells 61
Peptides, pacemaker regulation 12, 13, 17
Peripheral nervous system, HCN channels 36
Photoreceptors, HCN channels 35–36
Pindolol 104
Poincaré diagrams 61, 64–65
    bisoprolol study 67–68
    congestive heart failure 66–67
Posture 89
Potassium channels
    blockers, heart rate reduction 91
    HCN homology 30, 33–34
Potassium currents 3, 14
Practolol 104
Procoralan® see ivabradine
Propranolol 90
    atherogenesis effects 48–50
    clinical trials 103, 104
    ivabradine versus 84
Protein kinase A (PKA), pacemaker regulation 12, 17, 34
Psychosocial stress and atherogenesis 47–48
    β-blocker reduction 48–51
    endothelial dysfunction 50–51
Purkinje fibers 3

QRS complexes, ventricular pacing 38, 39

Repolarization, activation-induced changes 37–44
    atrial pacing 41–43
    ventricular pacing 38–41
Retina, HCN channels 35–36
RR intervals, heart rate variability 64, 65, 67

Serum lipids, heart rate effects 46
Signaling pathways
    adrenergic receptors 22, 24–25
    cAMP see cyclic AMP
    G proteins see G proteins

I_f current regulation 12, 14–15, 17–18
  nitric oxide *see* nitric oxide (NO)
Silent ischemia 69
Single HCN channel recording 7
Sinoatrial node (SAN)
  ablation, atherogenesis effects 45–47
  autonomic innervation 5–6, 61
  electrophysiology 61–62, 89, 90
  modulators 7–8, 16–17, 84, 91–93, 95
    see also specific drugs
  pacemaking activity 1, 3, 11, 37
    blocking 4
    HCN expression 9
    hyperpolarization-activated inward current *see* I_f current
    impulse initiation 37
    physiology 61–63
    repolarization and 37–44
    signaling pathways 17
    synchronization 62–63
  P cells 61
  T cells 61
Sinus bradycardia 61
Sinus tachycardia, hyperthyroidism 14, 15
Sotalol 103, 104
Specific bradycardic agents (SBA) 7–8, 16–17, 84, 91–93, 95
  safety and tolerability 78, 80, 84, 92
  see also individual agents
Staircase effect 86
Stress, atherogenesis role *see* psychosocial stress and atherogenesis
Stroke volume
  heart failure 87
  myocardial function 85
ST segment
  myocardial ischemia 55, 56
  time to 1-mm ST depression 77, 78–79, 81, 82, 83
Sudden cardiac death
  β-blocker trials 101, 102, 104
  heart rate link 1, 59, 103
    Framingham Heart Study 95
Sympathetic nervous system 5, 61
  glycoside effects 89
  heart rate acceleration 5, 87
    consequences 102
  signaling 17
Sympathomimetics, heart rate effects 56–58, 59
Sympathovagal balance, HRV as index 88–89

Tachyarrhythmias *see* arrhythmias
Tachycardia
  cardiovascular mortality and 95–98
  chronic effects 56, 85
  heart failure 56, 85, 93
  hyperthyroidism 14, 15, 18

Ta waves 41–43
T cells 61
Tedisamil 91
Thrombosis 72–73
    see also atherosclerosis; myocardial infarction
Thyroid hormones, I_f current regulation 14–15, 18
Timolol 103, 104
Treppe phenomenon 86
Triiodothyronine (T_3), I_f current regulation 14, 15
T wave alteration, ventricular pacing 38–41
    accumulation 38, 40
    angiotensin II role 40
    displacement 39, 40
    inversion 39

UL-FS49 *see* zatebradine

Vagal stimulation 5, 61
Vascular structure
    endothelial regulation 71
    heart rate effects 58–59
    luminal narrowing 69, 71
        see also atherosclerosis
    see also vasoconstriction; vasodilation
Vasoactive intestinal peptide (VIP), I_f current regulation 12, 13, 17
Vasoconstriction
    β-blockers 82
    myocardial ischemia 72
Vasodilation
    endothelium role 71
    myocardial ischemia 71–72
    nitric oxide role 72
Vasomotor dysfunction, ischemia 69
Ventricular fibrillation threshold 102
Ventricular myocytes
    action potential phases 89, 90
    developmental changes 21–22, 23, 26
    electrophysiological properties 25–26
    I_f currents 19–28
        adrenoceptor modulation 24–25
        human 25–26
        hypertensive rats (SHR) 19–21
Ventricular pacing
    angiotensin II role 40
    gene expression 40
    methods 37–38
    QRS complexes 38, 39
    T wave alteration 38–41

Zatebradine 7, 8, 91, 92
    ivabradine *versus* 16–17
ZD-7288 7